SUGAR BITCH

How I ditched the sugar and
ate my way out of obesity
and type 2 diabetes!

ROBERT ROYCE GALE

ROBERT ROYCE GALE

Sugar Bitch
How I Ditched the Sugar and Ate my Way Out of Obesity and Type 2 Diabetes

1st Edition, 1st printing 2021

Cover Concept Design and Interior Design: Steve Walters, Oxygen Publishing Inc.
Editor: Richard Tardiff
Author Photo: Kaitlyn Crossley

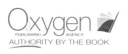

Independently Published by
Oxygen Publishing Inc.
Montreal, QC, Canada

www.oxygenpublishing.com
ISBN: 978-1-990093-17-3
Imprint: Independently published

SUGAR BITCH

ROBERT ROYCE GALE

DEDICATION

I dedicate this book to all who face this struggle with nutrition and health every day.

I hope my journey can be of help.

CONTENTS

PREFACE

It has been said that: "The illiterate of the 21st century will not be those who cannot read and write, but those who cannot learn, unlearn, and relearn."

- Alvin Toffler, 1970

We got fat

In 2016, more than 1.9 billion adults were overweight. Of these, over 650 million were obese.

We got sick

Death from diabetes increased by 70% globally between 2000 and 2019. In 2020, 463 million people worldwide suffered from diabetes, and it's estimated that it kills one person in the world every six seconds; that equated to 14,400 people a day, which is 5,256,000 deaths per year.

We are living in the Information Age, where we can attain information faster than we were ever able to do before. Even the data mentioned above, is only a click away on our smartphones, tablets or computers. Just as we can whip up those morbid worldwide statistics, the information leading to better health is also waiting to be accessed. How is it that there has never been more knowledge available, yet we are increasingly suffering from preventable diseases like type 2 diabetes? The information is out there, but unfortunately it's drowned out by the barrage of advertising for convenience junk food, and the plethora of quick-fix medications to treat these increasingly rampant diseases; online and on our TV screens.

Whenever you turn on your TV late at night, you can be rest assured that sponsored quick-fix pharmaceutical ads will be running. No matter what illness they claim to cure, these ads usually begin with a person wandering outside, happy and smiling, as the narrator tells us how great these marketed medications will make our lives. Then as we are nearing the end of the commercial, the narrator's soft, soothing voice begins running through the gamut of potential side effects and complications, ranging from headaches and flatulence, to the risk of blood clots and ultimately death. The last warning is to consult with your doctor to see if you are at risk. In America, The Food and Drug Administration (FDA) mandates that companies warn viewers of all the possible complications. If not, we might be lulled into a sense of wonderment. Luckily, hearing the many side effects is usually enough to make us second-guess the beautiful imagery.

What if fast food and junk-food commercials came with the same warnings? A melodic voice droning on about the many side effects from consuming a box of cookies might bring, informing us that ingesting multiple rows of them may lead to type 2 diabetes, insulin resistance and weight gain? Followed by the direst warning, "Consult your doctor if you have or you may be at higher risk of metabolic syndrome, as a steady diet of sweets can lead to complications such as a fatal condition... DEATH." Maybe if they listed these complications, it would make us think twice before consuming things that we associate as treats, and see them for what they are, a threat and a danger to our health and our well being.

It's time that we took a stand, and stopped gorging ourselves on the foods that are essentially killing us. We hold more power than we realize. Almost all cases of type 2 diabetes can be avoided by making lifestyle changes. Let's make these lifestyle changes sooner rather than later.

All it takes is for us to reduce our sugar consumption, and start eating our way out of disease with good whole foods that will fill us up. We can lower our blood sugar to normal levels and may be able to avoid, reduce or discontinue most medications. These are not fanciful claims; they are science-based facts.

Experts are fervently trying to get the message across.

Doctors and researchers are sounding the alarm about the hidden dangers of too much sugar, and the need to change how we eat. The Canadian Clinicians for Therapeutic Nutrition, created in 2017 and made up of about 3,500 physicians, believes sugar not dietary fat, is the primary driver of obesity and diabetes. The group wants to see Canada's Food Guide include guidelines favouring fewer carbs and more dietary fat. What's stopping us from taking their recommendations, making these switches and getting healthy?

It's confusing

There is so much marketing and conflicting information on what foods are good and bad for us. It leaves us wanting to say, forget it, let us eat what we want, and we'll take the meds!

It's hard to change

Convenience is tempting and easy. Taking medication is simpler than a lifestyle change. It takes a second to pop a pill while it takes time, self-control and dedication to change our lifestyle.

If these two excuses entered into your head as you read this, your next thought might be, why put yourself through the hard work of learning what is healthy, and eating better? Because the medications oftentimes treat the symptoms instead of treating the cause. The cause is your diet. By tackling the cause of your condition (an unhealthy diet), you will be freeing yourself of the daily worry and stress related to having a chronic disease. That reward will make life worth living.

Imagine controlling your choices, and gaining not only the healthy body you desire but a clearer mind as well. Once you bypass the excuses and take charge of what you put in your body, there will be no stopping you. And it can all begin with you accepting your reality the same way I had to accept mine many years ago...

INTRODUCTION

Best laid plans

My plan in 2009 was simple and not uncommon to many of us; to lose weight.

It should have been a no-brainer, a slam-dunk. It wasn't. My no-brainer plan ended up almost costing me my life.

It started innocently enough. My goal was just to drop a few pounds, maybe twenty.

I weighed 270 pounds, but at 6'2", 270 meant I was big but not huge. I just wanted to feel like myself again.

As a kid, then a teenager and in my early twenties, I had never been fat. I never had a six-pack or buff muscles, but I also had not stood out because of my size. I ate what I wanted played basketball every day, partied, and never gained much weight.

Once I entered my thirties that changed; the pounds began to pack on. By the time I was 51 in 2009, I felt I needed to address it, but I didn't overthink it. I looked at what I thought was the evident culprit; beer.

I'm a bar owner, and it's a given I'm always around alcohol and food. My daily go-to drink was beer, followed by a big meal.

I decided to adjust my habits; I swapped beer out for vodka. The change was motivated by the thought of reducing calories. I learned that one bottle of beer had about 150 calories, but a shot of vodka contained only half that amount. The solution? Drink vodka instead of beer; fewer calories.

I discovered that vodka with ruby red grapefruit juice cocktail is an excellent combination. I didn't look into the grapefruit juice cocktail's caloric or nutrient content because I didn't think it was relevant. Juice is good for you, right? It's full of vitamins and all sorts of healthful benefits. I felt I had added an extra fruit to my diet, just like our Canadian food guide asks us to.

My clothes soon became tight. My XL wardrobe had to be switched up to XXL, and sometimes the XXL felt tight. I wasn't losing; I was gaining. I refused to weigh myself. I was in denial. I was depressed and figured there wasn't much else I could do. So I ignored it. I drank my vodka cocktails, ate my heavy meals and pretended I was happy. Not realizing that soon, pretending would no longer be an option.

Gordito

I've technically been a very lucky man. I've been able to lead my life the way I choose (bad choices and good choices combined), and I've had the chance to travel where I want. One place that I always felt a pull to is Mexico. I've gone every year for the past thirty years. It has become an annual pilgrimage. I leave Quebec's cold winter and head down there for a few weeks of sun and fun, to unwind and forget about all my responsibilities. I always stay in the same hotel in the same small town.

December 2012 was no different. I'm in Mexico, but for the first time in thirty years, I can't unwind. I know something is frightfully wrong with me. I can feel it in every part of my body, even in my eyes. When I look in the mirror, I can see what my eyes are feeling. I'm sick...

It had begun on my first day in Mexico. I had been lying on the beach when a vendor came by with some coconut ice cream. I knew better than to buy from a beach vendor, but I bought some ice cream anyway. That evening I thought I had food poisoning. I had all the symptoms: diarrhea, light-headedness, nausea and an incredible thirst as if I was dehydrated. I didn't seek medical assistance, thinking it would pass. It didn't pass.

The next afternoon I still felt wretched. I was sitting at the bar near my hotel and contemplating what was wrong with me, as I watched Mexican women coming down from the mountains after delivering hammocks to other towns. These women are physically strong and robust, often carrying 40 pounds of hammocks on their heads to sell to the tourists. They looked healthy, something I am not, as I watched them.

One of those women is called Angela, a woman I've seen peddling her wares for years. I sometimes buy her a beer after she's done selling her hammocks. But due to our language barrier, Angela only speaks Spanish, and I know only enough Spanish to order food off a menu or call a cab, our exchanges stay pretty basic, and we are more along the lines of friendly acquaintances.

Angela never calls me by my name Rob; she refers to me as *Gordito*, meaning my cute fatty. Imagine you're not feeling positive about your body image, and you are known as... Gordito! It's a small town. We're talking about the type of place where you see the same expats hiding out from the winter, and the same locals year after year; everyone knows one another. And a bit like that bar in the hit TV show *Cheers*, where everyone would yell out "Norm" when he entered; wherever I would go in the town and Angela would spot me, she would yell out loud, "Mi Gordito!"

The first time she used it to describe me, I was embarrassed and didn't know how to react. It wasn't the first time I had felt conscious of my size, yet it was the first time I realized how much impact it was having. People stared. And I realized everyone was aware that I was indeed *Gordo*, overweight. She meant no harm by it, but every time our eyes would catch, I'd brace myself for her greeting.

But now I was sick and didn't have the energy to deal with seeing her and the greeting of "cute fatty." I returned to my hotel room. This was the worst I had ever felt. I was depleted of energy. I was craving sweet things to drink and a lot of them, sweating profusely, and my clothes were getting looser as if I was dropping weight. For the next week of my stay, I attempted to ignore all the symptoms (that spelled out diabetes) and tried to act like I was alright. It was a wasted effort. I couldn't even walk to the beach before I'd have to turn back due to fatigue. I departed for Montreal a few days before Christmas.

New Year, New Me?

On New Year's Day 2013, I had lunch with an old friend who is a nurse. and also happens to be a diabetic. I told her about my trip and what I initially believed was my bout of food poisoning. I confessed to her that I was worried that the supposed food poisoning symptoms were, in actuality, symptoms of diabetes.

To my surprise, and then fear, she offered to do a blood sugar test using her kit. I say fear because I didn't want to know. I had to know, but I didn't want to know. We went back to my house after lunch. I didn't bring the subject up, but she nonchalantly said, "Let's do it."

During the test, I just focussed on her face and eyes. I didn't look at what she was doing. I was looking for her reaction when she saw the reading on the blood-sugar tester. Her face went white, and I thought, "That's not good."

She turned the meter around, and it was blinking 26.8 mmol/L.

She confided to me that being a nurse and seeing a test so high, she had an obligation to call an ambulance, and have me taken to the nearest hospital. She said a reading so high could signal a hyper-glycemic emergency.

ROBERT ROYCE GALE

It was New Year's Day with most clinics closed and the hospitals filled to the brim. I told her I didn't want to go, but I promised to make an appointment with my doctor.

She left after I assured her a few times that I felt alright and just needed time to digest the news. I had to face the damage I had been doing to my body. I went and weighed myself. The scale indicated I was now 300 pounds. Confronting that I was that heavy was bad enough, but not as awful as having the number 26.8 still blinking in my mind. I needed to understand how bad a reading of 26.8 mmol/L was.

I googled everything I could about glucose levels. Normal blood glucose levels two hours after a meal for someone without diabetes is less than 7.8 mmol/L; for someone with diabetes, it should be less than 10 mmol/L. Suffice to say that my 26.8 mmol/L blood glucose level after my meal was extremely high and very dangerous.

I quickly moved from learning about glucose levels to information about diabetes. Listening to lectures and reading studies, and anything else that I could get my hands on about the disease. I read about the complications due to type 2 diabetes: amputation of toes and feet, dialysis, blindness from eye damage (Retinopathy), kidney damage (Nephropathy), stroke, heart attacks, nerve damage (Neuropathy), circulatory disease, high blood pressure, high blood serum, and dementia. I then googled the causes of type 2 diabetes. All the information pointed to sugar as one of the big bad guys.

It became evident that my diet was the problem. I thought of my failed weight loss plan a few years before, when I had replaced beer with vodka and grapefruit juice cocktail. I had only been concerned about the calories in the alcohol, and not even thinking about the sugar in the drink. I looked up ruby red grapefruit juice cocktail. It contains 28 grams of sugar in a 240 ml glass. 28 grams of sugar is equivalent to seven teaspoons of sugar per drink.

I thought of how many of those vodka cocktails I had in a day. How much sugar was I ingesting? I realized I was going through two, one and half-litre bottles every three days.

I was dumbfounded.

I had to have that talk. You know that talk when you look in the mirror, and you have to be honest with yourself? And there are always two questions. Do you want to live? Or do you want to keep on drinking and eating like this until you die? It will probably be a death afflicted with some of the horrors mentioned above.

There was no wiggle room. There was no magic solution.

I had to do something. And I had to make sure that whatever I did, it would stick. I didn't want a quick fix that left me heavier and unhealthy in the next few years.

I made a pact with myself that if I did figure this out, I would share how I accomplished it because if you can do something that everybody in the world doesn't think is possible, then it's your duty to share. I researched and researched, and then I set off on the plan that I thought would finally lead me to success, and it did!

Sounds easy, right?

The truth is it was far from easy. It's never easy when dealing with addiction and withdrawal, be it food, alcohol or drugs. It wasn't a walk in the park, but by having researched the information and planned out my steps, it was like I had a road map on how to get to my destination of becoming a metabolically healthier person.

Within a year of my resolution, I had lost 85 pounds and brought my sugar levels back to a normal range. I have now kept my sugar levels steady for over seven years. In 2020, I lost an additional 25 pounds to reach a total of a 110-pound weight loss. It, therefore, became my duty to share my road map.

My road map is in this book. Each of the chapters is devoted to my journey of knowledge, and the truths that I finally understood and incorporated into my life to become metabolically fit and lose weight. Achieving weight loss and long-term health doesn't have to be as over-complicated as we imagine. I am not, nor have I ever been, a complicated man. I like straightforward and easy. I wanted my book to be as simple and frank as possible. Within each chapter you'll come to understand the reasons I made each step, as well as the history of big business influence and its ties to supercilious research and policy. The real enemy is not our scale or our bodies, but decades of misinformation that has warped how we think about food. This book is about taking back our health, taking a stand against the lies we've been told about nutrition and fitness, and finally understanding what we need to do to be healthy. Will you take up the no sugar resolution and become a metabolic millionaire?

Chapter One
SWEET RESOLUTION

That fateful day when I resolved to "fix myself" is one that I will never forget. I was sitting in my comfy chair in my living room, on my iPad after my old friend had left, and I was a very scared, very angry overweight man. I called my sister and asked if we had diabetes in the family; nope came the answer. I knew at that point I couldn't blame anyone else for my uncontrolled blood sugar levels; it was self-inflicted. Right then and there, I decided to remove the one thing in my life that I knew did not benefit me long-term. I made a promise to myself that I would kick my sugar habit. My no sugar resolution can be seen as the first step on my road map.

Now the truth of the matter is that outside of the information I had googled that night, I knew incredibly little about my health or about the element I had just decided to kick out of my diet. If sugar was the big bad guy, how was I supposed to defeat this enemy (sugar) that I didn't fully understand? I read and read.

What is sugar?

Sugar, visualize that sweet stuff you keep in your pantry to add to your morning coffee or your next bake. Looks innocent enough, right? The sugar association boasts how it's an all-natural ingredient produced by plants, including fruits, vegetables and even nuts; and that is true. Sugar is the generic name for the chemical sucrose. Sucrose is produced during photosynthesis, where light converts water, carbon dioxide and minerals into oxygen and energy-rich compounds. All compounds created by photosynthesis are carbohydrates; therefore, sugar is a carbohydrate.

When we eat carbs, they provide energy to our bodies, but not all carbohydrates are created equal. There are simple carbs and complex carbs. A simple carb will have one to two molecules, while a complex carb will have three or more. When a carb has one or two molecules, it's absorbed quickly into our bloodstreams. Sugar being a simple carb with only two molecules, fructose and glucose, it's rapidly absorbed and creates spikes and dips in our blood sugar levels.

Our brain on sugar

Think of your body as an orchestra and all your body parts as the musicians. If each plays their part and plays it well, the result will be a beautiful piece of music. What if a wrong note is played and upsets the melody? The result might be a ruined symphony!

If our body is an orchestra, our music conductor is our nucleus accumbens, a region found in our brain. It's the conductor in the orchestra that determines what the music will sound like, by waving his wand and dictating to slow down or speed up the tempo. Similarly, our nucleus accumbens plays a pivotal role in the reward circuit of our brain, by determining if we want more or less of something. It's your nucleus accumbens that sends a message telling you "Mmm, that's good, let's have some more" or "No, I'm good, we can stop." Two neurotransmitters mostly impact our nucleus accumbens to decide on what message to send: dopamine, which is linked to desire and pleasure, and serotonin, which is linked to satiety and inhibition.

What happens to your body, to its delicate melody, its homeostasis, when you keep feeding it sugar? Sugar is a metabolic bully. Your body will access it immediately, and dopamine will hit your nucleus accumbens, transmitting a message saying, I WANT MORE! As you keep feeding it more, you begin to crave it and rely on having it. You may become addicted to it.

Studies have supported the idea of sugar addiction.

In a 2007 study in the journal Neuroscience Behavior Review, titled *Evidence for sugar addiction: Behavioral and neurochemical effects of intermittent, excessive sugar intake*, researchers asked whether or not sugar can be a substance of abuse, and lead to a natural form of addiction in rats. "Food addiction," the authors wrote, "seems plausible because brain pathways that evolved to respond to natural rewards are also activated by addictive drugs. Sugar is noteworthy as a substance that releases opioids and dopamine, and thus might be expected to have addictive potential." The evidence supported the hypothesis that under certain circumstances, rats can become sugar dependent.

The number of studies is endless, and many conclude the same message of possible sugar addiction.

In a 2018 study, *Sugar Addiction: From Evolution to Revolution* it's goal was to "analyze the important question of whether there is sufficient empirical evidence of sugar addiction, discussed within the broader context of food addiction." They tested this theory using an animal model. They concluded that "Finally, there is strong evidence of the existence of sugar addiction, both at preclinical and clinical level."

Robert Lustig, professor of Pediatrics at the University of California San Francisco, is a vocal opponent of sugar, adamantly broadcasting, without apology, that sugar is a "toxin."

Lustig authored *Sugar is the 'alcohol of the child', yet we let it dominate the breakfast table*; in January 2017 in The Guardian. He wrote, "when consumed chronically and at a high dose, fructose is similarly toxic and abused, unrelated to its calories or effects on weight. And that's why our children now get the diseases of alcohol (type 2 diabetes, fatty liver disease), without alcohol. Because sugar is the "alcohol of the child." He suggests that it's the amount of sugar consumed that is dangerous.

And North America is consuming large amounts of the sweet stuff, sometimes by choice, but frequently unaware that they are consuming it. The presence of added sugar is highest in the expected food products including candy, sweet bakery products and soft drinks. However it is also high in food products that many consumers choose as "healthy" options such as energy bars, cereals, sports drinks and juices. Why would someone purchase a healthy snack that has sugar as one of the ingredients? Simple, often sugar is hidden within processed foods, so people don't even realize they're eating it.

There are 56 common names that sugar in food goes by. Imagine 56 aliases! From the ones we recognize like glucose, brown sugar and cane sugar, to ones most of us would not recognize, such as sorghum syrup, treacle or galactose. (I have listed all the names for sugar at the end of the book.) Companies will often use liquid sweetener called high-fructose corn syrup (HFCS) which is derived from corn. In Canada, HFCS is listed as "glucose-fructose" in the ingredient list. Food manufacturers use HFCS because it's cheaper to use than table sugar, a quality preferred in many packaged foods today.

How much do you sugar?

The sugar that Canadians consume accounted for 21 percent of their daily calories in 2015, as per a 2015 Statistics Canada report, *Sugar consumption among Canadians of all ages*. On average, Canadians consumed the equivalent of 26 teaspoons of all sugars per day, be it from natural sources (such as the sugar in a piece of fruit) or added free sugars (such as the sugar in a piece of cake). It is estimated that over a third of those 26 teaspoons come from added sugars. Our American counterparts ingest 17 teaspoons of added sugar per day on top of the sugars found in natural sources. What is the recommended amount? The World Health Organization (WHO) recommends adults and children reduce their daily intake of free sugars to less than ten percent of their total energy uptake per day. A further reduction to below five percent or roughly 25 grams (six teaspoons) would provide additional health benefits. North Americans are way off the mark, opening us up to disease, addiction aand obesity.

Of course, most of us aren't trying to make ourselves sick and fat.

The problem lies in the vast amounts of sugar, declared and hidden (under aliases), that are put into various foods. In 2015 the American Centers for Disease Control examined 1,074 infant and toddler food products' nutritional information. It found that 32 percent of toddler dinners, the majority of child-orientated snacks and infant-aimed juices, contained at least one source of added sugar, with 35 percent of their calories coming from sugar. The amount of sugar we consume or feed to our children is hard to wrap our minds around.

I did a sugar audit. This was a big step two on my road map. I had already checked the sugar in my vodka concoction, but now I checked the amounts in the foods I consumed at home. Added up, the amount of sugar I was consuming daily, unbeknownst to myself was staggering. I was in a bind. I could easily abstain from adding sugar to my coffee, but how was I supposed to avoid all the hidden sugars in processed foods, to abide by my sugar resolution? It seemed like an impossible task, yet I knew I had to find a way.

ROBERT ROYCE GALE

Chapter Two
GO TO THE DOCTOR

I hadn't lied to my friend. I went to the doctor's the day after our rendezvous of the finger pricking blood sugar test, and my google frenzy of everything sugar. It can be seen as my step three on the road map. It's one I recommend to everyone and anyone who wants to get a handle on their health. Go to your doctor!

I didn't even bother making an appointment. I went to a walk-in clinic. Of course, that meant I couldn't see my general practitioner, but I was done with making excuses and pushing things back.

I told the attending doctor I was having tingly sensations in my toes, blurred and double vision at night and that I feared it was because I might be diabetic. He took my vitals and gave me a requisition for blood work. I went the same day to get it done. As much as I had left my health go for years, I now felt a pressure, a panic, to get it fixed. My doctor must have also felt the urgency of my plight; he called me to go in for an appointment only four days after I had gone for blood testing.

This appointment was about to change my life. I was apprehensive as I entered the room but anxious to understand where I stood regarding my health. He looked me in the eyes and told me I was diabetic.

My requisition for blood work had included a test called an A1c. It's a blood test that provides information about your average blood glucose levels over the past three months. It's used to diagnose type 2 diabetes and pre-diabetes. My three-month estimated blood glucose average was at 12.7 mmol/L. A non-diabetic would have a reading of less than 6 mmol/L. I was not a little diabetic, nor was I pre-diabetic. I was full-fledged, might lose a body part or my eyesight, diabetic; in other words, my diabetes was uncontrolled and dangerous.

My doctor immediately put me on Metformin, 2000 milligrams a day, and another medication called glyburide. He might have explained what they were for, but I was so freaked out by my diagnosis that I didn't remember the reasons. Once I got home from diligently having picked up the prescriptions at the pharmacy, I looked up what they were.

Metformin is the most commonly prescribed drug for diabetes. It reduces the amount of sugar released by the liver and improves how the body responds to insulin. Metformin seemed almost like a wonder drug. It puts little if any strain on the organs, doesn't cause weight gain, and comes with the added benefit of being the most affordable diabetes medication on the market. Glyburide lowers blood sugar by causing the release of your body's natural insulin.

Neither seemed to have many downsides except the frustrating part of knowing that I required them daily or else my health would suffer inexorably. That's a hard thing to accept.

I went onto the Canadian Diabetes Association's (CDA) website. One of the first things I read on the site was, "Type 2 diabetes can sometimes be managed with healthy eating and regular exercise alone, but may also require medications or insulin therapy." This was news to me. I didn't know there were people who didn't need medication to control their diabetes. Although I was resigned to the fact that I would never fully get off the pills, there was a glimmer of hope that maybe I could become one of those special cases that could manage my diabetes, if I stuck to a healthy diet with no sugar. Heck! At the very least I wanted to attempt to lower the doses.

Bloody morning

Aside from the medications, I had also picked up my first testing kit. When you have type 2 diabetes, you need to test your blood glucose levels every morning. It's a little nick on the finger, not a big deal unless you're squeamish and afraid of the sight of blood. I am, and I hated the idea of having to do it, but again, I was resigned to the fact that this was now part of my daily life routine.

The next morning, I woke up and headed to my kitchen to test my blood. I got my kit out and attempted to prick my finger. I was scared, and I guess I didn't stab it hard enough because there was only a little trickle that came out, not enough to get a reading. I pricked a different finger, nope. The third time had me trying to squeeze blood out of, yet again, a not deep enough nick, resulting in another false reading. By the end of it, I had ten jabs on different fingers, my hands were all bloody, and I was hot and dizzy. I had to sit down before I fell down. I felt dejected. I knew I had to figure out how to do it properly, but it was so hard. I kept thinking I will have to do this every day for the rest of my life. And not only that, but I will also have to take the meds for the rest of my life. The discouragement was palpable.

I kept thinking back to what I had read on the CDA site. Could I somehow not only lower my doses, but go a step further and reverse my diabetes by eliminating all consumption of sugar, and removing the need for these daily pricks? The only problem was that after having learned how sugar was in everything, I knew how challenging eliminating sugar was going to be.

Withdrawal

I made a monumental change. This can be identified as my fourth step on the road map. I cut out all ultra-processed foods and drinks, everywhere that sugar could hide. The first month off of ultra-processed foods and alcohol was a nightmare. I had been slugging back 10 to 12 drinks a day for more years than I cared to remember. I probably had never gone more than a week without a drink since I was 15.

Like my alcohol consumption, my diet also had stayed the same for the last 40 years or so. I liked my convenience food, my easy take-out meals and large quantities of everything delicious.

I was going through withdrawal. Omitting both alcohol and ultra-processed foods brought on feelings of irritability, depression and even anger. There was no way for me to know which symptoms were associated with which withdrawal. I was a mess. I felt physically terrible, had constant headaches, was sweating profusely and had cravings. The worst was the cravings, the moments at night where you would give almost anything to have something sweet. I didn't give in, and had decided that no matter how disgustingly bad I felt, I wouldn't. I knew it was going to get better. All my reading had told me that it would, and I held on to that belief.

Chapter Three
ROSETTA-LIKE SCIENCE

I was hungry at night; not having snacks was a killer. The removal of all my bad food habits meant I had to find some way to occupy my time, so I wouldn't be thinking about the foods I couldn't consume. This would be step five on my road map; find ways to keep busy and not be at a loose end. I started to play Scrabble online to keep my hands and my mind occupied. Scrabble has always been there for me. In 1985 I had moved down to Los Angeles to become a comedian. It wasn't a perfect time in my life. I had come to realize that making it as a comedian would not only be incredibly difficult but also might not make me happy. I was broke and felt stuck, unable to leave. That's where Scrabble stepped in. I got on the Scrabble game show and won a cash prize! That money allowed me to come home. And now, when my withdrawal symptoms were hitting the hardest, Scrabble was there once again to save the day. I played up to 25 games online simultaneously to keep busy. It helped me avoid those nighttime temptations.

Of course, a man cannot occupy himself with Scrabble alone. I also started following the Rosetta Mission, a spacecraft on a 10-year historic mission to catch up to a comet and manoeuvre a landing. I began tracking it online. The comet was travelling at 36 thousand miles an hour, and the team on Earth sent a signal to the rocket to drop a probe on it the size of a washing machine.

I remember thinking, how incredible are we as human beings, to design, propel and accomplish this bit of space marvel technology?

Imagine the diverse groups of international participants, businesses and governments involved. Imagine the technological compromise between minds to get this project off the ground?

My next thought went straight to, if we have the great minds to accomplish this venture, how do we not have the great minds to fix our health? In the last 90 years or so, we've become obese and metabolically sick here on Earth, without any genuine conviction to alleviate the problem.

We now live in a world of misinformation, a lack of a Rosetta-like science to curb and then eliminate obesity, which in turn would lessen the likelihood of many diseases and extend life. Why?

How did we, over the years, become big sugar's bitch?

Believe it or not, we had begun on the right foot towards healthier nutrition using processed foods at the end of the 19th century. Processed food is any food that has been altered during its preparation, be it as simple as canning, dehydrating, freezing or baking. One such example of a processed food done right at its inception was the humble cornflake.

The story goes that in 1894 John Harvey Kellogg accidentally left some boiled maize out one night, and it went stale. He passed it through some rollers and baked it, creating the world's first cornflake. Now, John Harvey Kellogg was a doctor and a nutritionist, and he proclaimed that his breakfast food with no added sugar was the perfect healthy, ready-to-eat morning meal. That healthy ready-to-eat cereal was unfortunately not the one produced by the Kellogg's company owned by his brother Will. The two brothers had gotten into a conflict; John wanted to keep the cereal pure for its health benefits, while Will wanted to add sugar to the flakes to make them more palatable to the mass market.

Soon after the creation of the cornflake, the American government began pushing breakfast as the most important meal of the day (just the energy needed to work those long, tedious hours at the farm or the factory). The U.S. Department of Agriculture (USDA) promoted it by publishing the food guide, *How to Select Foods*, in 1917. It was the follow-up from a guide created a year earlier in 1916, *Food for Young Children*, which classified foods in five categories: milk and meat, cereals, vegetables and fruits, fats and fatty foods, and sugars and sugary foods. Consequently, the population followed the two guides' recommendations and began eating more fruits, vegetables, milk, and more sugar. Sugar "serves as fuel for the body and to flavor the food," the manual affirms. "Unless small amounts of very sweet materials, sugar itself, syrup or honey are used, the diet is likely to be lacking in it." The two guides were not the first to believe and promote the properties of sugar. But the food guide solidified the stance of the importance of sugar as nutrition.

Accessibility and taste leaped forward in the 1920s when Clarence Birdseye, seen as the father of frozen foods and inventor of the double belt freezer, introduced non-local foods to the masses, that tasted as fresh on the day they were plucked from the soil or pulled from the lakes and seas.

Had processed food been limited to canned green beans or frozen peas and fish, we might have been better off, but of course it did not. The creation of easily accessible, sometimes delicious yet incredibly unhealthy foods ensued, aka ultra-processed foods. We're talking about those fun foods that have added ingredients such as sugar, salt, fat, artificial colours and preservatives. Popsicles came out in 1924 and 1927 saw the arrival of Hostess cakes and Kool-Aid on store shelves.

Government, scientists, and convenience were changing our diets. And we were eating it up. For the next 30 years, the list of unhealthy foods grew and grew, as did our accessibility to it. Better machinery, a new variety of crops and livestock, coupled with new pesticides and improved irrigation methods, meant farmers could offer their products at a lower cost. Advances in transportation, food preservation, and home storage such as fridges and freezers in almost all homes began to equalize local food availability. We could keep a quart of ice cream in our freezer or a bag of milk in our fridge!

Getting the produce to people was becoming easier as well. Roadways and the interstate were connecting people. Now consumers had readily available food off the shelf, or cut up at the butcher at affordable prices.

There was no going back. The world had changed from simple plain fare confectioned at home with the barest of ingredients and reliance on seasonal produce and, of course, the ability of the cook in the 1900s kitchen, to a smorgasbord amount of cheap options for the taste buds, be it nutritious or junk-filled ready-made frozen meals, snacks and desserts. It must have felt like the world was an open oyster of edible choices for the entire population. What a time to be alive and not worry about something as silly as food determining your health! I sighed heavily. That was not my reality. My eyes were open to the harm these foods had done to me.

Chapter Four
SENDING US DOWN THE WRONG PATH

Not a big shocker here, but outside of Rosetta, Scrabble and way too many walks to mention, the thing that kept me busy was reading. I wanted to learn as much as I could about nutrition. And as I read, I got more intrigued about how we as a society make the food choices we do. I knew that I had certain assumptions about foods that lingered since my childhood. Those assumptions, at times, had dictated my choices. Such as how fruit juice was healthy (hence the debacle of gorging myself with it during my years of grapefruit and vodka), but it wasn't the only erroneous assumption I had. I don't know about you, but for years I associated fat with an unhealthy diet. Thinking that butter, cheese, and other fat sources I consumed were slowly killing me, by clogging my arteries and adding pounds to my waistline. How had this become a mainstream doctrine in our society?

Ancel Keys - Mr. Cholesterol

Many of the so-called healthy processed foods we consume today, be it low-fat mayonnaise, non-fat yogurt or our plentiful pasta dishes, can be traced back to the research that Ancel Benjamin Keys completed. He was an American physiologist who studied the influence of diet on health.

His first big accomplishment came at the request of the American government. They asked the physiologist to create emergency meals for their parachute troops in 1939 as the Second World War was beginning. Ancel Keys took up the challenge and went shopping. The result of his shopping excursion, combined with his knowledge of what soldiers would require as emergency nutrition, was the K-ration, a high-calorie simple lightweight meal that included sugar tablets, candy, chewing gum and cigarettes as some of its ingredients. They were such a success that by 1941 America had adopted it as their standard field ration, feeding these high sugar K-rations to all their combat soldiers. You might be asking yourself, how is the inventor of K-rations responsible for non-fat yogurt?

All for heart health

Ancel Keys hadn't expected K-rations to be used as standard fare for combat soldiers, creating the emergency high-calorie high sugar pack and its misuse seemed to stir his interest into starvation research, and the best way to rehabilitate Second World War victims. He began a study with 36 men who had volunteered to starve for six months and then re-nourished for three months. It was seen as a groundbreaking study, which brought forth many results, such as the importance of nutrition research and how diet directly affects the mind and the body's functions. The study suggested that diet could significantly affect blood pressure, cholesterol level, and resting heart rate. His findings were detailed in the publication *Biology of Human Starvation*.

The ball was rolling.

Having already established the importance of diet in our body's function, he decided to study the connection further. In 1946, he noticed an increasing amount of deaths due to heart attacks in the

United States. He conducted a study to see what was causing this increase and if it was diet-related.

He observed 286 middle-aged businessmen in Minnesota and concluded that those who suffered heart attacks had higher cholesterol levels. Keys proposed the theory that this buildup of cholesterol was due to fat consumption. He believed that fats (the fat from meat and dairy products), was the culprit in the rise of heart attacks, rather than what was being considered by other researchers; ageing, stress and an increase in cigarette smoking. It was way too small a study to make such heady conclusions, but it didn't seem to stop Keys from making them. The meat and dairy industries did not take kindly to his theory and criticized it and him harshly.

Taking the show on the road

His follow-up study to prove his fat culprit theory was the controversial Seven Countries Study in 1958. In this study, more than 12,500 middle-aged men from seven countries, Italy, Greece, Yugoslavia, Finland, Netherlands, Japan and the United States were followed.

Keys initially looked at 22 countries for fat intake and heart disease.

He was accused of cherry-picking these seven countries out of the 22 as they had the strongest correlation between saturated fat intake and heart disease. He seemed to conveniently leave out countries like France and Germany, where they consumed a lot of saturated fat, but didn't have a lot of heart disease or obesity.

Some unanswered questions exist in the study to this day.

For example, the rate of coronary events in Eastern Finland was three times higher than in Western Finland despite identical diets and lifestyles. Similarly, the inhabitants of Corfu consumed less saturated fats than their countrymen in Crete, yet coronary heart disease was higher in Corfu. But Ancel Keys chose not to address those concerns, and instead decided to use the study's findings to strengthen his diet-heart hypothesis, and promote a diet he created called the Mediterranean diet. He wrote three diet books on it.

In its simplest form, the diet-heart hypothesis states that people should eat less cholesterol and saturated fat to reduce cholesterol and heart attacks. The Mediterranean diet favours that hypothesis by emphasizing fruits, vegetables, pasta, and olive oil, with only small portions of meat and dairy products allowed.

The media and government didn't take long to publicize the findings to the population, and the population in turn, ate it up!

Keys made the cover of Time Magazine on January 13, 1961. Time labelled him "Mr. Cholesterol," quoting his advice to cut insidious dietary fat from 40 percent of total calories down to 15 percent.

Keys only demonstrated an association of fat and heart health, yet that association would become the basis for America's food guidelines targeting saturated fat as the "bad" foods. The food guidelines became the basis for the food pyramid in America. The logic was to reduce fat/ saturated fat consumption based on certain percentages. One could eat 33 percent made up of bread, rice, potatoes, pasta, and other starchy foods; fruit and vegetables for another 33 percent; milk and dairy foods for 15 percent; meat, fish, eggs, beans, and other non-dairy sources of protein at 12 percent, and the remaining eight percent from foods and drinks high in fat and/or sugar.

It seemed as if every American government entity jumped on board the low-fat train. The American Heart Association (AHA) correlated eating fat with what they dubbed the coronary heart disease epidemic. The National Heart, Lung, and Blood Institute put out a large campaign to promote low-fat diets. The National Cholesterol Education Program and the National Institutes of Health also supported a low-fat, high-carbohydrate diet. Even the

American Senate Select Committee on Nutrition and Human Needs highly recommended that Americans reduce their total saturated fat consumption.

Don't think that Canada didn't join the low-fat train as well. Canada's Guidelines for Healthy Eating in 1990, a companion publication from Health Canada, suggested that Canadians "choose low-fat dairy products, lean meats, and foods prepared with little or no fat" while enjoying a variety of foods.

Food items such as whole fat milk, whole eggs, and red meat had become almost taboo since they were thought to increase the risk of coronary heart disease. Consumers were left searching for replacements.

Enter the introduction of low-fat, higher carbohydrate food products. Food companies had a heyday, churning out these supposedly heart-healthy and health-conscious low-fat products disguised as food. But who would want to eat them? Cardboard tasting is often the term used to describe those early low-fat offerings. The solution was simple; add more sugar. The sugar barons lined up in support of the diet-heart hypothesis, and who could blame them? They were about to have a serious payday. What better ingredient to replace natural fat in processed foods than yummy sweet sugar?

In 1988, the AHA began a program to label foods to promote healthy options. If a food had a "heart healthy" seal of approval, it meant the consumer was supposedly making a healthy choice. By 1997, over 600 products were certified and labelled with that seal of approval, including Kellogg's Frosted Flakes, Fruity Marshmallow Krispies, and Low-Fat Pop-Tarts. It begs the question, had the government and its programs become so trapped in the idea of low-fat being heart-healthy, that sugar-laden refined high-calorie foods were being sold to the population with a stamp of healthy approval?

The Seven Country study had concluded that serum cholesterol was a risk for coronary heart disease, but that blood pressure, diabetes and smoking were also risk factors. Why were we neglecting the other risk factors?

Why had Keys' research and push for a low-fat society gone seemingly unchallenged? Why had governments and companies taken his word as law, and not researched the dangers of the fat replacements they were proposing in our diets, such as margarine, and of course, the increase of sweeteners?

We are a society known for testing and retesting theories; that's how we had landed on the moon, put a probe on a comet, and even created the atomic bomb! Yet with one researcher's word, the world seemed to bow down to the low-fat ideology. Or had there been challengers, and governments refused to listen to them? And was I harming or helping myself by not removing fat from my diet?

Chapter Five

PASS THE BEEF

I couldn't contemplate removing animal protein and fat from my diet. I mean, at this point I was eating no processed anything, no sugar and trying to stick to whole real foods. Taking fat and meat out would leave me with some gnarly lettuce leaves, and a sure-fire chance of falling back to my old ways. I refused to do that.

Step six of my road map; eat foods that fill me up and keep meals interesting. If my body couldn't have its usual sugar and liquor dose, I had to feed it things that it would enjoy and be satiated by. I knew I needed a basic food plan to follow.

I would begin my day with bacon, two eggs, a fruit, and a small glass of freshly squeezed orange juice. I decided to have the same breakfast every day. I loved it and figured it would make life easier to stick to my plan. For lunch, I had the luck of having a great restaurant right by my bar. For years it's been where I've gone to eat. The chef has a knack for making everything taste amazing. Before my resolution, I would head over for one of his heavier on the menu stick-to-your-bones-type meals. I knew I couldn't have those anymore. I asked him if he would be willing to make me a special daily lunch menu that fit into my plan, and that would be nutritious and delicious. Did I mention how lucky I was and how super talented he is? He said yes, and made me these wonderful lunches that respected my food restrictions. It awakened my tastebuds to veggies, and introduced produce I would never have thought of if left to my own devices. My supper at home was simpler fare. It would be a protein, be it steak, fish or chicken, a veggie and a starch, typically new potatoes. It was mostly clean eats, and I was mostly happy with it. For the first time in a long time, I found a diet that I could stick to and would maybe give me a chance to heal myself.

I couldn't give credence even for a second that reducing fat and bringing in sugar was healthier. I didn't trust that Ancel Keys had gotten it right. I knew I wasn't alone. Many disagreed with him and his concept of fat being the all-out evil in diet and health. They thought that the governments' low-fat, high-carb strategies would lead the world to become unhealthier, fatter and maybe even put heart health at stake. They spoke out. Some were ridiculed, others dismissed, but it's worth noting that they were not lightweights in the field; they were physiologists, biochemists and doctors. They had also compiled data, completed studies and brought out interesting and valid arguments to the discussion of nutrition and health.

The challengers

John Yudkin was a British physiologist, nutritionist and author of more than half a dozen books. He was one of the first to challenge Keys' conclusions. He believed that sugar, not fat, was the cause of illnesses such as obesity, heart disease and diabetes; a belief he had put forward since 1957. He was highly respected in the field of nutrition until he went against the low-fat movement, and then the sugar industry tore him to shreds. It all came to a head with his controversial book called *Pure, White and Deadly* (1972). In this book, he theorized that when it came to diet, the blame for bad health should fall squarely on the shoulders of sugar. In it, he went so far as to oppose Keys and the diet-heart hypothesis, by inquiring if there was any causal link at all between fat and heart disease, or if it was accidental. In the last chapter, *Attack is the best defence* in the latest edition of *Pure, White and Deadly,* it lists several examples of the sugar industry's attempts to coerce and interfere with Yudkin's research and message. And how when those attempts failed, they resorted to attacks and lies, such as the World Sugar Research Organisation (WRSO) publishing articles under titles such as 'For your dustbin' in which they refer to his book as "science fiction." The WRSO was forced to print a retraction after Yudkin took the matter to court. Yudkin didn't stop there. He detailed how the British Food Foundation (primarily sponsored by sugar refiners) went on the attack to discredit his work, and attempted to silence him by pressuring boards and committees not to select him as a member. How conferences he was a designated speaker would be cancelled (once under pressure by Coca-Cola), when he refused to temper his message about the dangers of sugar. Also, he addressed how Ancel Keys' attempted to discredit his work through unjust claims, falsehoods and personal smears such as referring to him as "absurd."

Doctor George Mann also felt that Keys' evidence did not support the diet-heart hypothesis. Mann, a respected nutritional biochemist, researcher and physician at Vanderbilt University, had conducted field studies in the 1960s and 1970s in Africa intended to disprove Keys' theory. He recorded that nomads who consumed high-calorie diets rich in saturated fat had very low blood cholesterol levels. He had many back-and-forths with Ancel Keys and many others over this study. In the arguments Keys attempted to poke holes in Mann's research. It can be seen as an attempt to besmirch his work. One peer even went so far as to label Mann a "heretic." Mann addressed these claims in a published article where he states, "I am not a heretic, I am a scientist." Lower down in the article, he adds, "diet/heart enthusiasts who, by their noisy propaganda hope to coddle and prolong the diet/heart hypothesis. That hypothesis has been shown wrong by scientific method. I believe that because I believe in the scientific method." After he retired from medicine, Mann declared the diet-heart hypothesis to be "the greatest health scam of the century."

Over the years, many more researchers had issues with the diet-heart hypothesis and the attempt of the government to cut the fat, such as Dr. Edward H. Ahrens Jr. He criticized a government effort to reduce consumption of cholesterol drastically, saying it treated people as though they were "a homogeneous group of Sprague-Dawley rats." (Because of their uniformity, such rats are ideal for research). The list goes on.

I could write a whole book on the challengers and those who believed in the hypothesis, but what good would that do? It won't change the simple fact that there's a problem, and after years of non-fat yogurt and cereals for breakfast, that problem has not appeared to diminish.

I can't tell you which scientist was right or wrong. I can, though, provide you with the fact that in America, where the diet-heart hypothesis gained popularity first, Americans today are 70 percent more likely to die from heart disease than they were in the 1970s, when the diet-heart hypothesis took hold.

A Public Health Agency of Canada 2018 report revealed, "Heart disease is the leading cause of death globally. In 2015, an estimated 8.9 million people died from heart disease, which represent 45 percent of all non-communicable disease deaths worldwide. In addition, heart disease is the leading cause of disability-adjusted life years (DALYs), lost due to ill-health, disability or early death worldwide."

Those are scary statistics. It can't just have been fat in our diet that has caused this amount of death and unhealthiness. If so, shouldn't the rate of heart attack have lowered with every package of low-fat delight?

There has been a pushback against the belief that fat is bad in the last few years, a movement to embrace fats in all their glory. Yet, even with the pushback, there aren't many of us who can state the diet-heart hypothesis hasn't warped our thinking. You might not be aware of it, but the years of advertising low-fat products, and government campaigns on the importance of reducing our fat intake, have shaped our thinking. It made us believe that having eggs daily for breakfast will heighten our cholesterol levels, or that having a piece of bacon will clog our arteries and bring us that one step closer to death. Yet, we don't think twice about ingesting our toast and muffins. They are just fibre that will fill us up, and maybe if we eat too many of them, we might gain a few pounds, right? Isn't it odd how we see sugar as something that might make us gain weight, but we don't correlate it with health and death? Why do we give sugar a pass when there are studies and proof that sugar can kill?

ROBERT ROYCE GALE

Chapter Six

SUGAR MONEY,
THE ROOT OF ALL CAVITIES

I had waded through so much conflicting information as I read the research. It did keep my mind off snacking, so that was a positive, but it was distressing to read. I didn't understand the governments' reaction; a total lack of response to sugar studies while the diet-heart hypothesis had sparked whole advertisement campaigns. Why had governments in the very least entertained the notion that sugar might be detrimental to our health, as so many studies had concluded? I was stumped.

Why had sugar gotten a pass?

Sugar had shifted into an essential part of the social fabric of our lives. It's a beloved staple, right? Reward children with sweets; if they eat their veggies, they get dessert. The concept that veggies' health benefits are far more important than the deleterious effects of excess sugar has become ingrained in our minds. We see sugar as just empty, harmless calories.

Why would we have thought sugar was harmless? Simple, we believed in our government, and our government sent us that message. The real question is, why were governments so invested in this message? The answer to that question appears to be straightforward - money!

Sugar makes governments and companies a whole lot of money.

According to the International Sugar Organization website, "Currently, about 110 countries produce sugar from either cane or beet, and eight countries produce sugar from both cane and beet." That's 110 governments invested in keeping sugar sales and production high. The global market for sugar and sweeteners totalled about $77.5 billion in 2012. Sugar is a multi-billion dollar business. And that is before we discuss the amount of money that companies make, once they process that sugar and create all those darling foods we love to purchase.

For all food production, it might amaze you to know that ten companies hold 90 percent of the market: Nestlé, PepsiCo, Coca-Cola, Unilever, Danone, General Mills, Kellogg's, Mars, Associated British Foods, and Mondelez. And, of course, those ten companies make billions and billions of dollars; a lot of invested interest in the status quo of you not worrying about your sugar consumption.

How has this very profitable industry wound its way to ensuring we don't see sugar as unsafe for consumption? They created the boards that look into it, and give politicians a lot of money regardless of their political leaning, as long as they looked favourably towards the sugar industry. They also control the studies by financing them and at times paying the scientists large sums to get their desired results.

A revealing 2016 study in the JAMA Internal Medicine, titled *Sugar Industry and Coronary Heart Disease Research: A Historical Analysis of Internal Industry Documents*, examined Sugar Research Foundation's internal documents, historical reports, and statements relevant to early debates, about the dietary causes of cardio-vascular heart disease.

One of the documents in that report showed that a trade group called the SR (Sugar Association) paid three Harvard scientists to publish a 1967 review of sugar, fat, and heart disease research.

Unfortunately, it isn't only in the past. With a quick google, you can find many more examples of how the sugar industry and those ten production companies fund and control many of the studies that downplay sugar's role in our health. Exasperating to think that it would be allowed, that we, the people, would allow it. It's like having a compulsive gambler responsible for shuffling the cards at the poker table. Would you trust the outcome? Of course not! Yet we allow the gambler at the table because we want to play; ditto for sugar.

We love it, and yes, we crave it, so we allow ourselves to be fooled by governments and companies into believing that it isn't harmful. When we get cavities, it isn't because of the juice and candy we eat; it's because we don't brush enough. We gain weight; it's because we're lazy, and we don't move enough. We buy pedometers to get our steps in and refuse to control what we put in our mouths, even rewarding our hard workouts with carbs; we must replenish our bodies' energy! We tone out the message of reducing our consumption by scientists and doctors, because we enjoy the sweet taste on our tongue as we let the bitter truth of its noxious effects slip through our fingers.

It might sound like I am demonizing the sugar industry and, by extension, sugar itself. Make no mistake, I am. I needed to because it helped me stay focused on my plan. Sugar is a temptation for most of us, but for me, it is also an addiction. To give in by saying, "one cookie or soda won't hurt" would put me at risk. It would be a slippery slope back down. If I slipped and fell back into my old ways, there were chances that I wouldn't stop on the ground, but end up six feet under it! The other part of this was that it wasn't difficult to demonize the sugar industry. The paper trail of corruption is well documented, as are the disturbing diseases associated with over-consumption. They might not get enough coverage, but the information is out there for all to see.

ROBERT ROYCE GALE

The problems our sweet tooth brings

A couple of extra pounds on the waistline doesn't seem like that big a deal. Not a real problem right, but unfortunately that bigger waistline is actually one of the symptoms of something called metabolic syndrome. It's also known as insulin resistance syndrome, or the cooler expression syndrome X. MetS is your body's way of telling you you're headed in a bad direction. MetS is like rolling on the highway to hell. It's a pre-diabetic state; it's a pre-obese state. It's not an illness, but rather a cluster of conditions that increase the risk of heart disease, stroke, type 2 diabetes, fatty liver and an endless list of other medical disorders.

The cluster conditions include high blood pressure, insulin resistance, excess body fat around the waist, and abnormal cholesterol or triglyceride levels. You can have one of these conditions (be it a bigger waistline, high cholesterol or whatnot) and not have metabolic syndrome, but it does mean that you have a higher risk of disease. Take insulin resistance; in people who suffer this, their cells don't typically respond to insulin, and glucose can't enter into the cells. Insulin is the hormone made by the pancreas that helps sugar enter cells to be used as fuel or energy. As a result of being insulin resistant, your blood sugar levels rise even as your body churns out more insulin to lower your blood sugar. The link from having uncontrollable blood sugar to type 2 diabetes is a pretty straightforward one. Being insulin resistant has put you at a higher chance of developing diabetes. And if you combine more of these conditions, your chance of bigger complications rises inexorably.

MetS is increasingly common, and up to one-third of American and Canadian adults have it, leading to a society that is laden with chronic ailments. Outside of the evident large waistline, there are not many visible signs of having MetS. You can't see high cholesterol, a fatty liver, or high blood sugar. But you can feel the effects of diabetes, such as increased thirst and urination, fatigue, and blurred vision.

Sound familiar? Those were many of my symptoms, as well as the visual factor of having a larger belly. This is the problem of my sweet tooth, my being a bitch to sugar, had gotten me. I wanted to reverse the roles. I wanted to make sugar my bitch and take away its power over my life. I wanted to go from having metabolic syndrome to becoming a metabolic millionaire; healthy and carefree!

ROBERT ROYCE GALE

Chapter Seven

WHO WANTS TO BE METABOLIC MILLIONAIRE?

Metabolic millionaire is a term I made up while I'd been thinking about my long-term goals. My main if very hopeful goal, was to stop being diabetic or at least to be a healthier diabetic.

I knew that my new diet to attain that goal, would also bring weight loss. Now, of course, I wanted weight loss, but it was never my main objective. If it had been, I think I would have failed in my mission. I would have fallen into the trap that many of us do. Many of us yo yo with our weight because we become lax once we lose a few pounds, our purpose having been achieved and no longer deemed necessary.

I didn't want short-term weight loss. I wanted long-term health, combined with being a healthy weight. This is where metabolic millionaire came to be. The chances of becoming a millionaire are near to one percent worldwide. The odds of keeping to a substantial weight loss over nine years are also about one percent. Hence my goal had the same odds as that of me becoming incredibly financially wealthy. Dollar signs were not what I was after, though. I wanted to be health-wealthy; a metabolic millionaire!

To do so, I knew I had to stick to my plan. I had to make consistency step seven of my road map. I didn't aim to be consistent only with my food choices, but also consistent with my habits. I ate my meals at the same time every day. I'm a routine-oriented person anyway. Even when I was unhealthy, I followed a daily schedule of unhealthy choices (beer at 7 pm with a large meal following, mixed drinks with pizza and hours of tv at night). Without a new routine of planned meals and habits, I knew that I would feel lost, and my old habits would creep back in. I wanted to avoid that like the plague.

I wasn't following a specific commercial popular diet. Any commercial diet can make a person lose weight if they follow them, be it the Keto diet, Mediterranean diet, the South Beach diet, grapefruit diet or any other of the kazillion diets out there. The two issues I had with following a commercial diet, was that most diets are centred on weight loss and not health gain, and I also didn't want to stifle myself with their specific rules and dietary restrictions. I couldn't picture myself counting calories or points, peeing on a test strip to see if I was in or out of ketosis, or checking to see if it was a high-carb day or low-carb day. That sounded stressful to me, and hard to maintain.

In the first month, I hadn't thought of my eating in terms of low-carb. Rather I was aiming for consistency with my meal choices, and those choices so happened to have been low in carbohydrates. Once you omit all the added sugar, oddly, you also omit a whole lot of carbs. My plan (let's nickname it the eat-to-heal-Rob diet) was simple, and only had a few rules; no added sugar, no ultra-processed foods, eat at preset times and only eat a predetermined amount (a single serving, no going back for a second helping). I didn't cut starchy vegetables or remove fruits or anything else that might be considered drastic. I had included two cheat treats a week, a serving of sugar-free ice cream to give myself something to look forward to. Even in my cheat treat, I had kept to my sugarless plan, and amazingly, it was also low-carb. As I entered the second month, I realized that eliminating sugar and eating low-carb went hand in hand.

Living la Vida low-carb

There's no official guideline that defines what comprises a low-carb diet, but the accepted norm is any diet that limits your carbohydrates to less than 100 grams a day, is deemed a low-carb diet. I'd take it a step further and suggest that any diet that reduces your carbohydrates from your normal consumption is technically a low-carb diet for you. The question remains; is it the right type of plan. For myself, the clincher was not seeing it as about weight loss, but about considering my personal health conditions, MetS and type 2 diabetes. The studies correlating a reduction of these conditions with low-carb diets are very persuasive.

A study titled *Dietary carbohydrate restriction improves metabolic syndrome independent of weight loss* published by the journal JCI Insight in June 2019 examined which type of diet, be it low, moderate or high carbohydrates, helped adults who had MetS. Their findings concluded that "... MetS can be rapidly (within 4 weeks) reversed by an LC diet in the majority of participants who are obese even when one of the main characteristics of the syndrome, increased waist circumference/adiposity, is locked out of the equation."

A motivating conclusion when you consider that one of the main downfalls when changing eating habits is that we don't see the point because we don't think we're having the right result (weight loss). This study demonstrated how even if your weight doesn't change, your health can improve immensely in a short a time period of time; as little as four weeks!

A 2014 study titled *Low carbohydrate diet to achieve weight loss and improve HbA1c in type 2 diabetes and pre-diabetes: experience from one general practice*, by David Urwin, concluded that "... the majority of patients lose weight rapidly and fairly easily; predictably the HbA1c levels are not far behind. Cholesterol levels, liver enzymes and BP levels all improved. " Their study had consisted of observing 19 type 2 diabetes and pre-diabetes patients over an eight month period. Out of the 18 (one of the 19 having dropped out at the beginning), only two patients remained in the abnormal range of blood pressure, and all 18 had substantial weight loss.

The more studies I read, the more I felt that low-carb was the evident answer for helping me treat my ailments. On top of that, it wasn't as if the idea of using them to treat health conditions was an untested fandangle concept. Low-carbohydrate diets are far from new to the world.

The first person that flirted with the idea of a low-carb diet for treating those who have type 2 diabetes was John Rollo. John Rollo was a Scottish military surgeon. He was highly respected in the medical community for his work in diabetes studies, and was often consulted about cases. In 1797 he published *Notes of a Diabetic Case*, which reported on the results of treating two diabetic Army officers with a low-carbohydrate, high-fat and high meat diet. The use of a definite diet for diabetic patients was revolutionary. What struck me was the diet that Rollo had proposed was not only a low-carb diet but was also high-fat. Could the high-fat component be important?

As the first few months of 2013 passed, and I had removed my high carb-filled meals in exchange for moderate protein and whole lower carbs, something glorious had happened. My cravings had begun to diminish. I did not search wildly for the next sweet thing to put in my gullet. The troubling part was that although I wasn't searching for sweet things, it didn't mean that I was feeling full. I often felt hungry. Sometimes the hunger pangs would go away after I drank a few glasses of water, but other times, the feeling stayed. I began to wonder what I could do to help reduce the pangs, and the idea of low-carb high-fat began to swirl in my head...

Chapter Eight
TWEAK IT

Forever can be a scary word. Forever is a big commitment and those big commitments make us take a step back and say, are we really ready for this? I didn't want to commit to forever with my plan. I still don't. Imagine feeling stuck in anything "forever," it's daunting. My step eight on the road map was to resolve not to veer off my diet for a short, yet long period of three months. It would permit the switches I had made to my lifestyle to reach their full impact, by letting my body get used to the new foods and habits. I told myself if it wasn't working, I could tweak the plan at that time or switch it fully. Thinking of it as only a three-month commitment gave me strength, by seeing an end date if it sucked...

Saying it sucked was an understatement. It was 90 days of hanging on by my fingernails, trying to stay hopeful and not cheat. Completely changing my lifestyle was incredibly challenging, and I doubted myself all the time. As I got closer to the three-month deadline, my doubts strengthened, even as the cravings began to lessen. I wondered if I was doing it all for nothing. I had ostracized myself socially (drinking alcohol and eating-out are two very big social activities), and it felt as if my goal was still so far away. I felt alone in my struggle.

When I felt close to my lowest, that's when my sister sent me a video by Dr. Peter Attia. He is a Canadian physician focusing on the applied science of longevity. The video was his 2013 TED Talk, *Is the*

Obesity Crisis Hiding a Bigger Problem? Peter Attia's approach in the TED Talk was candid, and he admitted to his past faults and errors. He spoke about the need to investigate further the relationship between insulin resistance, obesity, and diabetes. The TED Talk began with him admitting that in 2006 he had held a patient in the ER "in bitter contempt," judging her for being a severe diabetic and requiring a leg amputation. He said, "As I looked down at her in the bed, I thought to myself, if you just tried caring even a little bit, you wouldn't be in this situation at this moment…" I was taken aback to hear a doctor admit that he had these thoughts! His honesty enthralled me. What came next surprised me more; this doctor, who looked like the epitome of good health, admitted that only three short years later after having judged that patient, he himself, had developed MetS and become insulin resistant. He realized how "Despite exercising three or four hours every single day, and following the food pyramid to the letter, I'd gained a lot of weight …"

He explained how he "…became almost maniacally obsessed in trying to understand the real relationship between obesity and insulin resistance." As I finished watching the video, the feeling of being alone in this mission towards good health had disappeared. Here was a doctor, who was also searching for the answers for his patients as well as for himself. The kicker was that he seemed to have found them. His results of reversing his insulin resistance encouraged me. I found myself clicking on and listening to more of his podcasts.

One of them explained his thoughts on ketogenic diets and attaining ketosis, a state where your body burns fat for fuel instead of sugar. He also wrote many articles on this subject, as well as many more on varied commentaries of experiments with his health. He had taken self-experimentation a notch higher than I could ever contemplate, by doing full-on medical tests at his home. Attia had a centrifuge in his house. A centrifuge is a machine used typically to separate fluids of different densities. He could take his blood every 30 minutes, spin it in the centrifuge, and see what changes were taking place every hour. (I remember thinking he must have a very understanding wife, because he admitted that his fridge would be full of urine and blood samples half the time.)

It changed my outlook. I began seeing my quest for health as an experiment. And as all experiments require, it was now time to evaluate the results as my third month was up.

I was proud I had stayed the course but unsure if it was working. I wanted proof. I headed to the clinic in mid-April and asked if I could have my blood work done. I wanted to see if my blood sugar levels were still off.

When the results came back, I was floored: 5.7 mmol/L on my A1c! I had lowered it by seven points. The reading put me at the level of non-diabetic. The eat-to-heal-Rob diet had more than worked. Since I was doing so well, I decided to stick with my plan for another 90 days, without any major dietary changes. That isn't to say I wasn't exploring how I could improve it. It had been 90 days of hanging on by my fingernails... and there was also the nagging issue of continuous hunger. I wanted to find a solution to the problem, and felt that the research on high-fat diets would lead me to some answers.

Let's add a smidge of fat?

I took the quick skip and a hop from investigating low-carb eating, to low-carb high-fat (LCHF) eating. One of the game-changers was when I read low-carb high-fat advocate Gary Taubes' book *Good Calories, Bad Calories*. Gary Taubes is a staunch believer in the low-carb movement, and in the book, he argues that refined carbohydrates contribute to many chronic ailments. I had associated sugar with diseases, but had never fully comprehended the role that refined carbs like flour might play in my ailments. Taubes explains that the key to good health is the kind of calories we take in, not the number. He also links eating fat to weight loss and the elimination of hunger. I quickly realized how beneficial it would be to throw in some extra healthy fats, such as an avocado every day.

Another handy addition came when I read Dr. Steve Phinney and Jeff Volek's *The Art and Science of Low Carbohydrate Living*. In this book, Dr. Phinney recommended adding some sodium and potassium back into our diets. By adhering to my eating plan, I had cut out my sodium intake by a ton (it's shocking how much sodium they put in processed foods). I had begun suffering from dizzy spells and feeling a little off; I decided to give his recommendation a try by adding chicken broth to my supper. It did the trick, and soon my dizzy spells were a thing of the past.

Caryn Zinn, Amy Rush and Rebecca Johnson, in 2018, concluded that a well-planned LCHF meal plan could be considered micronutrient complete, dispelling the myth that an LCHF eating plan is suboptimal in their micronutrient supply. Their study, *Assessing the nutrient intake of a low-carbohydrate, high-fat (LCHF) diet: a hypothetical case study design*, was published in BMJ Open. The study concluded that, "Considering this way of eating provides a replete set of nutrients and has been shown to be effective for improving metabolic health, particularly for people with diabetes, it should at least be considered a suitable dietary option for populations." The major critic of LCHF meal planning is that there may be a lack of complete nutrients. The study noticed a small lack of iron, but not anything else.

There are many similarities when you go through the different popular LCHF diets. Sure their carb gram allotments change depending on the diet (from as low as 20 grams to as high as 150 grams!), but most of them stick with the same similarities, such as higher fat content and very little to no sugar. I don't recommend one diet plan over another because I don't believe there's a one size fits all answer to what, when and how people should eat. No two people are alike, or need the same optimum amount of carbohydrates they should be ingesting. It's about trial and error, self-experimentation and evaluating your results. There is no other way to identify if a plan is working or healthy for you.

My experimentation had led me to embrace LCHF eating. My mindset had switched from thinking of my diet as reducing basically everything, to seeing the importance of the quality of the food I put in my mouth. I began making a conscious effort to incorporate healthy fats, such as nuts and those previously mentioned avocadoes. I also began to check the number of carbohydrates I consumed. I found my sweet spot for carb consumption was around 50 grams. The rest of my diet stayed the same, yet soon my hunger pangs were a thing of the past.

ROBERT ROYCE GALE

Chapter Nine

EFFICIENCY EXPERT

One of the most boring words on the planet must be accountability. It reeks of responsible behaviour, and frankly, of dullness, but it's also crucial to attaining success. Accountability is inconvenient as it gets in the way of all our short-term pleasures and distractions. Without accountability, it's easy to get sidetracked by social media, TV, or sometimes even by sleep, instead of concentrating on our goals. We delay the work that we had set out to do that day, preferring the fun or the mind-numbing, and the day passes us swiftly by without accomplishing the tasks.

I wanted success, so I had to bite the bullet and keep track of my actions, to ensure I got them done. So, Step nine on my road map, I kept a journal. It helped me continue to see this plan as an experiment. Taking notes made it seem more clinical, and made me feel like I had to give it my all to keep my results legitimate.

I used nothing fancy or electronic for my journal, just a regular old-school spiral notepad in robin egg blue, one that you can even pick up at a Dollar store. You would think writing notes down about your day would be tedious. At least, that's what I had thought before I did it, but I was wrong. My journal became an highly effective motivational tool.

I found it satisfying to jot down my daily fasting glucose levels and the exercises I completed. I loved seeing the days add up on paper. And yes, exercise was part of my equation for success.

Exercise is recommended for all type 2 diabetic patients. The Diabetes Canada website states that, "Over the long term, exercise can result in:

- Improved fitness and body composition.

- Reduced complications of diabetes such as lowered risk of heart disease.

- Improved diabetes, including blood sugar, blood fats, and blood pressure.

- Improved overall fitness and health."

All good things; I wanted to work out and have all these happen to me. Through the research I completed, I learned that high-intensity interval training (HIIT) held many benefits. The study, *Low-volume high-intensity interval training reduces hyperglycemia and increases muscle mitochondrial capacity in patients with type 2 diabetes* published Dec 1, 2011, concluded that, "Two weeks of low-volume HIT, involving only 30 min of vigorous exercise within a total time commitment of 75 min./week, lowered 24-h average blood glucose concentration, reduced postmeal blood glucose excursions, and increased markers of skeletal muscle mitochondrial capacity in individuals with T2D."

I was intrigued with trying HIIT. The promise of requiring only 30 minutes of exercise a couple of times a week was a big selling point. I am, at my core, a pretty lazy man, although I do prefer thinking of it as being an efficiency expert, someone who likes to get the maximum result for the minimum effort. I saw 30 minutes of effort as a great fit for my maximum-minimum philosophy.

Unfortunately, the idea of high-intensity training or even regular training was one that felt out of reach. Exercise, when you are obese, feels almost as hard as controlling your food cravings. You want to do it, but it's hard. I had no cardio. I was weak and felt out of breath easily. I was not well enough to begin a high-impact, high-intensity program. I settled on completing a walk per day. In the beginning, those walks zapped all of my energy. I was diligent and made it a goal not to miss one. When the temperatures plummeted to -30 degrees Celsius, whether it was snowing or in the early spring raining, I fought to overcome all my instincts to retreat and get inside where it was comfortable. I knew I could reverse the effects of years of drinking and overeating if I just kept at it. I recorded the distance I covered daily down in my journal.

Slowly but surely, I began to feel stronger. I wanted to push myself more, and I began adding speed walking intervals in my walks. I saw it as my beginning of interval training.

As I was nearing the sixth month of my journey, I tinkered with the idea of adding bodyweight exercises to the mix. I had lost a lot of weight but also a lot of muscle. I needed to begin getting some of that muscle tone back.

I was very fortunate to have stumbled upon the work of Mark Sisson. Mark Sisson is a fitness author, a former distance runner, a triathlete, and Ironman competitor. This man knows fitness! Although he stressed the importance of high-intensity interval training, such as sprinting to achieve results in his blog's webpage *Mark's Daily Apple,* he also addressed the importance of varied training and putting the fun back into fitness. On his website, he writes, "... it seems the diet and exercise industry today is calibrated toward exactly that; the idea that you need to struggle and suffer to drop excess body fat, achieve fitness goals, and be 'healthy.' My most prominent motivator is the pursuit of pleasure and happiness in my life."

The idea of pleasure and happiness in this process was a new one for me but one I fully welcomed. Sisson endorsed play, "The important thing is to take the edge off, so make the decision right now to incorporate play into your healthy lifestyle."

I got my basketball out. I decided I would include basketball into my newly minted bodyweight program, and headed off to the outdoor court. I'd do a few bodyweight exercises such as push-ups, sit-ups and squats, and then I'd finish with some hoops. I had always hated gym-type workouts because I found them dull. It's hard to motivate yourself to do something when you see it as drudgery, but when I added basketball to my training, it became a pleasure to go workout.

Even though I had incorporated shooting some hoops, which could be considered as cardio, I still kept up my walks. They had become a sort of therapy, a period of my day where I could reflect. It also didn't hurt that we were approaching summer, and the weather was making it a lot more enjoyable to go out for my strolls.

As the sun stayed out longer, my journal pages multiplied and showed me that I was on the right path. Since I had been recording my daily fasting blood glucose levels, it was easy to check and see that I was on a pattern of controlling my levels. I didn't have wild sugar spikes, and I felt better than I had in years. I was excited to get my blood work done now that my second three-month increment had passed. I headed off to the clinic in July.

Once in my doctor's office, I advised him about my additional bodyweight workout routine. He then gave me my blood test results. My A1c came back at 5.5 mmol/L, completely normal. I smiled inside. I was doing this; I was fixing my health! My doctor also informed me he was changing my Glyburide prescription to Onglyza. I was totally uninterested in his reason for the switch of the pill. I just nodded yes. My only thought was I want to get off of them all.

Chapter Ten

DOING BIG THINGS

After my last doctor's visit, I was feeling good. He had weighed me at the appointment. I had reached a milestone of 75-pound weight loss, and yes, I had accomplished that in only seven and a half months. Put that with the A1c results; I was flying high as a kite.

My transformation was becoming evident; gone were my feelings of being far from reaching my goals or hanging by my fingernails. In their place, confidence was building. One place where my weight loss was apparent was my wardrobe.

My clothes were fitting loosely. Luckily over the years, I had not thrown out garments as I had gained weight. I still had all my large size shirts from my twenties, and those are what I was wearing. I did have to go splurge on a pair of new sweatpants. It was done for decency's sake. I didn't want to moon people when I headed out to the court for my workouts in ill-fitting pants.

My friends and customers were remarking on my physical and mental changes. My outlook had brightened and I loved sharing the information I had learned about health. I was more optimistic than I had been in years.

One of my friends told me I should contact a reporter named June Thompson from *The Montreal Gazette*, the number one English language newspaper in Quebec. The reporter had a recurring health column, and was always on the look out for people taking charge of their health. My first thought was that would be neat, and the next was why not try? I sent her an email explaining my journey. She responded quickly and told me she wanted to feature me in an upcoming article. She sent out a photographer, but our interview was done over the phone.

The article appeared in the paper only a short week later, July 29. Seeing my picture in the newspaper spurred me on to keep learning, and tweaking my diet and exercise routine. It became another tool to hold myself accountable; after being in the paper, I vowed I wouldn't regress and go back to how I was before.

I wasn't tempted to go back to the old me either way. The feeling of being able to do so much more than I had in years was incredible. You don't realize how much being overweight and unhealthy tires you out. Carrying all those extra pounds is hard on your joints, and now that I didn't have the burden of the weight, I felt light and springy. I did one switch to my diet. I had learned that potatoes were considered a high-glycemic vegetable, and I decided to try to remove them from my diet. To transition from eating them, I ate the skin for a few weeks without the center. After a while I realized I wasn't yearning for them anymore. I had successfully weaned myself off potatoes. The summer continued on a high note, and by September I had lost another 10 pounds. My next scheduled doctor's appointment was set for the new year, and for the first time in my journey, I didn't feel the need to prove that my plan was working by hitting up the clinic earlier. I had the evidence. I had surpassed what I thought I would be capable of attaining in less than a year; 85-pound weight loss, gobs of energy and controlled fasting sugar levels.

HIIT 'em up

I ran into a friend at a restaurant I hadn't seen for a while, and he was surprised by how striking my weight loss was. I told him about my workout regimen, and how my only issue was that it was getting a little cold to exercise outside. His eyes brightened, and he divulged that his son-in-law had just opened a gym right underneath my dentist's office.

I had a scheduled dentist's appointment the week after, and I told him I would stop in.

The gym was small and thankfully didn't give out that feeling of the 1970s meathead vibe that I must confess I had always associated with gyms. I signed up for three high-intensity 30-minute sessions weekly after talking to the owner, my friend's son-in-law. He dispelled every perception I had of personal trainers. I liked his style and how he spoke up about health and training. He was down-to-earth yet very knowledgeable.

Although I had felt comfortable upon my first visit to the gym, I still scheduled private training sessions during the hours the gym would be less busy. I was apprehensive about what I'd be able to do, and how others would perceive me. I shouldn't have had those worries. No one stared at me. HIIT was unlike anything else I had ever done. It was quick and intense. I was completely sore after my first workout. By the third week I was still sore, but had gotten used to the pace and the exercises.

Stopping the popping

I had entrenched myself in reading and listening to podcasts at nights and had found myself going back to one specific person, a Canadian doctor named Jason Fung. I had listened to his talk on insulin toxicity and found his arguments very compelling. He planted the seed that this disease (type 2 diabetes) was curable without drugs. I began questioning if my A1c was normal because of the switches I had made in my diet, or because I was on the medication.

I wrote to Doctor Fung and told him my story, diagnosis, weight loss, A1c results, and my wish to stop taking the drugs. He emailed me back and affirmed that with my A1c levels at 5.5 mmol/L, I was in the normal range and could be considered not diabetic.

This in turn gave me the courage to try eliminating the medication. I told myself I could always restart if I noticed a rise in my fasting blood glucose levels.

November 18 was the first day that I reduced my medication, by taking out the Onglyza pill. I had decided to remove it before the Metformin. By mid-December, I was off both pills and had not seen a change in my morning fasting blood glucose levels.

Looking back, I should have also talked to my doctor beforehand. It's important to consult a physician whenever making such a significant change, especially if you are on any other medications. In a way, I didn't because I didn't want him to caution me against it. Also, I was on no other pills outside of my diabetes pills, so I wasn't worried about the effects of removing or lowering the doses would have on other medications. I didn't feel bad, lightheaded or sick after stopping them. I felt free. I hoped my one-year appointment with my doctor would provide me with the assurance that I had made the right choice.

Chapter Eleven
ONE-YEAR ANNIVERSARY

I had decided I would head out to Mexico in the New Year instead of in December. I would go after the Super Bowl and after my doctor's appointment. January 2014 was the first anniversary of beginning my sugar resolution; the doc visit followed by the trip in February would be like the cherry on top of my sugar-free sundae.

The changes that had happened in a year were incredible, and I was excited to get my results from the doctor. I had asked him to do a complete lipid profile on me as well as my A1c. I wanted all the tests, because I wanted to see how all of the results connected with one another, and compare them as I continued with my health experiment. As I got to the office, my excitement, as well as my anxiety had heightened. I was anxious to hear what he thought of my stopping the meds. What if my results showed that I needed the medication again, or the doctor felt I had put my health at risk by quitting and wanted me to restart taking them?

My doctor welcomed me in and greeted me with a big smile on his face. He began with the basic yearly check-up protocol. He weighed me: 215 pounds. He checked my pressure and reflexes, normal. He chuckled as he called me "the poster boy" for what to do when you have diabetes.

As we sat down to discuss the blood results, I let the cat out of the bag. I told him I had stopped taking my meds. December 21, 2013, being the last day that I had taken a Metformin pill. I explained how and why, and told him I had monitored my fasting blood glucose levels since I had gotten off the meds. He said, alright, and then stared at his paper. I gathered I had surprised him, but he didn't say I was wrong for having done it. Although I'm sure he would have preferred that I had consulted with him first.

He began with my A1c. It was at an average of 5.5 mmol/L. Normal. I was ecstatic as he continued. It felt like I was eagerly awaiting my report card after spending an entire school semester studying hard and doing extra credits. The next test was my lipid profile.

A lipid profile is like a metabolic report card. It gives you a baseline to really understand where you stand in regards to your health. It is known by a slew of different names Coronary Risk Panel, Lipid Panel, Fasting Lipid Panel, Non-fasting Lipid Panel, Cholesterol Panel, or Lipid Test. But at the end of the day, no matter what name it goes by, it does one simple thing, it measures the lipids (fats) in your blood. You will usually have four results on your lipid profile. Your level for:

- Low-density lipoprotein (LDL) cholesterol

- High-density lipoprotein (HDL) cholesterol

- Triglycerides

- Total cholesterol level (HDL+LDL+20% Triglycerides=Total cholesterol level)

Cholesterol is part fat and part protein. Just hearing the word cholesterol sometimes gets us apprehensive, our minds jumping straight to heart attacks. Although its reputation is well earned as an artery clogger, cholesterol is also required in our bodies as it's essential to many metabolic processes. Think of cholesterol as little couriers that travel through the bloodstream to deliver essential packages to help our cells grow.

Sometimes doctors will do only a single test for total cholesterol and not a full lipid profile. The more extensive the lipid profile you get, the more you can use it to compare down the road. That's why when people ask me what test they should request, I advise them to ask their doctors to do the full lipid profile test from the get-go. With all the advancements happening in science and the testing available, you might as well get as complete a screening of your metabolic health as possible.

Why are the results of this test so significant?

If the lipids measured do not fall into the recommended ranges, you might be more at risk for heart disease. It might also mean that you have MetS, as abnormal cholesterol levels and high triglycerides are two of the conditions linked with MetS. The results are some of your very important metabolic markers.

- LDL can lead to clogging of the arteries. Think of the fat in the LDL as super sticky and clinging to the blood vessels' walls; the more of it you have on the walls, the narrower the passage becomes. Essentially you want it low.

- HDL picks up the excess cholesterol and carries it to the liver for recycling. Think of it as a vacuum, cleaning your blood arteries. When it's at healthy levels in your blood, it can reduce your risk of heart disease, heart attack, and stroke. In other words, you want it high.

- Triglycerides are the fats from the foods we eat. Think of them as storage units for the extra calories we consume that hang around in our bloodstream. They are the most common type of fat in our body. High levels of triglycerides are linked to liver and pancreas problems. Elevated triglycerides also increase the tendency of blood clotting. You want it low.

My results all fell into the average healthy range. I couldn't keep the grin off my face. I imagine it must be hard for people who haven't ever had health issues, to understand how good it feels to be told you are average and normal.

Back in a little town in Mexico

The grin stayed on my face as I boarded the plane and arrived in Mexico. As soon as I checked in, I set off to go by the water. I was about to do something I hadn't done in years. I walked on the beach with my shirt off. For years before 2014, I had been too self-conscious to even think of removing my shirt. My shame of being fat had kept me from enjoying the simplest of pleasures, the feel of the sun on my skin. Now that I had dropped the weight, there was nothing that was going to hold me back. I was doing my HIIT training on the beach and taking long walks. I was not concerned if I would tire out, my body would ache or worried how people would perceive me. When the locals and the regular snowbirds saw me, they were gobsmacked, amazed at my one-year transformation. One of my favourite moments was when Angela laid her eyes on me. She smiled and called me "mi Flaquito," my skinny boy. Flacco in Spanish means skinny. I told her, "No mas Gordito, yo Flaquito." It translates to no more cute fatty, I'm a skinny boy!

I felt I had not only figured it out, but had gotten to a place where I could easily maintain my results. I knew what snacks I could have, how to work out efficiently and keep myself in check, or so I thought…

Chapter Twelve
2 FAST 2 FEAST

If my journey had been made into a movie, receiving the doctor's results confirming that my plan had worked, and that I didn't require medication for my diabetes, would have been the end scene. It would have been that or when Angela sweetly referred to me as Flaquito. But my life is not a movie, and things never wrap up as neatly as they do on the big screen. I had accomplished my goal to lose weight and get off the meds, but soon I noticed my weight was creeping back up. That wasn't part of the plan. I knew that between 83-90% of people who lose large amounts of weight gain it all back within two years. I thought I had figured it all out, that I wouldn't fall into that trap and was doing everything right. Yet, I must have messed up somewhere because the pounds were coming back on. I racked my brain to figure out what I was doing wrong. I hadn't added back sugar, nor had I changed my meals. Or had I?

A false sense of confidence

I scrutinized my diet. Had I made any switches? The answer was an unfortunate yes. When I began my bodyweight exercises around the sixth month mark, I had incorporated a clean snack to curb my hunger and give me a quick boost of energy. That clean snack was almonds. I would eat a bunch of them twice a day. I loved almonds, and they worked well since they gave me something crunchy and hearty to chew. The only negative to them was that they were an expensive snack. So when I was shopping at my local big box store a few months into the new year, and saw a big 1.3 kg container of mixed nuts for the low price of $22, I thought what a steal, and bought a few containers in reserve for my snacks!

Now my usual almonds were plain, no salt, sometimes roasted, but that's as fancy as it would get. The container of mixed nuts was salted. I figured that a little bit of sodium and a variety of different nuts wouldn't hurt me or my pocketbook. I opened the container soon as I got home and took a handful of them. They were delicious, peanuts, cashews, pistachios, all kinds of goodness. I took some more...

I finished the first container in three days. I was in denial about the amount I was consuming, and kept sneaking into the kitchen for a quick handful. Aware that a hefty 1.3 kg container should last me way longer than three days, I began putting the nuts in pre-portioned baggies to stop myself from eating too many. The plan was a baggy per day. On Tuesday, I was already eating Friday's baggy. As March was rolling in, my clothes were fitting tighter again. No buttons were popping, but I felt the material stretching where before it had hung comfortably loose. It was a subtle difference, and I ignored it until the end of the month. I knew I must have gained a couple of pounds, but I didn't figure anything major. I stepped on the scale and realized my weight gain was nearing 15 pounds. After months of successfully keeping to an 85-pound weight loss, I had made a nasty dent in my results.

I couldn't handle having the big container of nuts in my kitchen or my home. I was mad at myself for being so stupid. Nuts are healthy snacks if you don't overdo them. A few of them go a long way in satisfying you, so why was I over-consuming them? They tasted good, I loved the salt and the nuttiness combined, and my nucleus accumbens must have been sending out the "oh, let's have more of those" signal. But I didn't require the large amount I was ingesting, and my body was turning it into glutinous fat on my frame.

My only option was to ditch the mixed nuts, and go back to the more expensive, slightly less yummy, but easier to stick to portions of prepackaged almonds.

I also wanted to find a way to help me drop the extra 15 pounds I had gained; removing the nuts would surely stop the weight gain, but I wanted to drop the rest. I hadn't lost any weight since September. My diet and exercise were all about maintenance, and I needed a little push to get the pounds off.

I turned once again to Doctor Fung. Doctor Fung was an avid believer in intermittent fasting for weight loss. He literally wrote the book on it, *The Complete Guide to Fasting: Heal Your Body Through Intermittent, Alternate-Day, and Extended Fasting*. Fasting appeared to be based on some good science with many studies to prove it. I decided I would give it a try.

So you starved yourself?

No, not at all. Starvation is harmful; it's suffering and involuntary. Intermittent fasting is controlled cycles of brief periods of fasting and periods of unrestricted eating. You should feel in charge of the process at all times. Intermittent fasting's roots are derived from traditional fasting, a universal, age-old ritual used for health or spiritual benefit.

Lately, fasting for weight loss has captured the public's imagination. Some are intrigued; others are worried it will head to nefarious effects on the body. A misconception of intermittent fasting is that it will lead to a slower metabolism and weight gain in the long run. It's erroneous because humans can tolerate up to 48 hours without food with no ill effects on their metabolisms. On Jason Fung's website, *The Fasting Method*, he has a breakdown of why fasting helps. "At its very core, intermittent fasting simply allows the body to use its stored sources of energy - blood sugar and body fat. This is an entirely normal process and humans have evolved these storage forms of food energy precisely so that we can fast for hours or days without detrimental health consequences. Blood sugar and body fat is merely stored food energy to fuel the body when food is not readily available. By fasting, we are lowering blood sugar and body fat by using them precisely for the reason we store them."

There are many ways to introduce intermittent fasting into our lifestyle. It's relatively easy to do because it isn't a dietary intervention that restricts or chooses which foods to eat, but rather when you should eat them. We already "fast" daily while we sleep. Intermittent fasting can be as simple as continuing that fast a little longer after we wake up. There are a few methods of intermittent fasting that are more well known. They include:

- Time-restricted eating; in this approach you have set fasting and eating windows. An example of time-restricted eating is the 16/8 method, where you fast for 16 hours a day and eat only during the remaining 8-hour window.

- Alternate-day fasting, also known as Eat-Stop-Eat, alternates between fasting days and days of no food restrictions. Example: Monday, Wednesday, and Friday are fasting days, while Tuesday, Thursday, Saturday and Sunday have no food restrictions.

- Whole-day fasting, for example, the 5:2 diet, comprises of five days with no restrictions, while the remaining two days you consume only 500 calories per day.

The Harvard School of Public Health in 2017 wrote, "A systematic review of 40 studies found that intermittent fasting was effective for weight loss, with a typical loss of 7-11 pounds over 10 weeks." They did caution that "It would also not be appropriate for those with conditions that require food at regular intervals due to metabolic changes caused by their medications, such as with diabetes." A lot of the information I found warned that if a person is underweight (BMI < 18.5), pregnant, breastfeeding, or under 18, they should not undertake intermittent fasting. It also warned that those who take prescription meds, suffer from gout or any other serious medical conditions would require medical supervision during fasting.

I wasn't on any medication and no longer had any medical conditions. I decided to try to fast for one meal, one day a week. It was a test to see how my body felt doing it. One day a week, I would skip breakfast; eat at noon, snack, and then supper at 6 pm. In three months, I had lost the 15 pounds, but I had also realized I hated not having my breakfast. I decided to switch and follow the 16/8 method of intermittent fasting. I ate in a window from 10 am to 6 pm while fasting the rest of the day. It allowed me to keep my breakfast but reap the benefits of fasting. I rewrote to Doctor Fung to give him an update about my health and my experience with intermittent fasting.

From: Rob Gale

Date: March 22, 2015 at 12:08:47 PM EDT

Subject: Fwd.: weight loss update

Hi Dr. Fung,

Thought I would give you an update on my health.

After successfully losing 85 pounds and reversing my DM2 in the first year, it was brought to my attention that between 83-90% of people who lose large amounts of weight actually gain it all back within 2 years.

They call this the "honeymoon period" of weight loss, and I really wanted to avoid this as much as possible. But even with this knowledge, my weight crept up 15 pounds just after the one-year mark. I decided to try intermittent fasting one day a week, and within 3 months, I had lost all the weight I gained.

I have been off my meds for over one year, and my recent blood work indicated an A1c of 5.6

Blood pressure is now at 120/80, and TG and HDL-C are normal.

Chapter Thirteen

THE MANY PITFALLS OF LIFE

When I had my first weight gain in 2014, I thought, oh boy, here I went and messed up, but it won't happen again!

This is me being completely honest. It did happen again and again...

Every year for the first few years, like clockwork, I would gain some weight back; some years it was as little as eight pounds, other years as much as 28. My saving grace was that I continued to do my every three-month self-evaluation. It allowed me to catch myself each time and figure out what I was messing up. The first year it was the nuts. Second, my portions had gotten bigger. In the third year, I had tried to put a particular high-glycemic food back into my diet, and the fourth, believe it or not too many tuna melt sandwiches had gotten into the mix. In each of those instances, I had made excuses as to why I was consuming these items. Either calling it testing to see if my metabolism could handle it or smudging the amount of my portions, telling myself it's the foods I'm allowed so a little more won't hurt. I knew each and every time it was wrong, so why was I caught in this continuous cycle?

Gary Taubes uses this one quote in almost all his talks and his interviews; the quote is by Nobel Laureate Richard Feynman, "The first principle of science is you must not fool yourself, and you're the easiest person to fool." Fooling myself was exactly what I was doing. Why did I feel a need to trick myself, because irrationally I wanted my excuses to be true? I wanted to indulge and do things that in the long run would harm my body. I was lying to myself for emotional reasons instead of analyzing my choices scientifically. I had learned what my tolerance was for carbohydrates and high-glycemic foods. These were not things I needed to try and incorporate more of into my diet. Doing so was irrational, as was consuming larger portions. I didn't require them. By taking my emotional, irrational wants out of it, I could see the truth in the science; the truth my body wanted me to accept. In a way, my self-evaluations were the safety net that also allowed me to fudge my plan. Because I would fool myself knowing I'd catch myself later. It was time I stopped playing the fool.

I knew what worked for my body. I had to pursue my plan and not get sidetracked by the bumps in the road trying to derail me. If not, I would always be stuck struggling to find my happy balance in life. From 2017 on, I took a clearer view of my nutrition. Before adding any dietary inclusions, I reflected on whether the particular item was something my body needed, or just a capricious want. It stopped the yearly weight gain. Quitting being a fool was a big step 10 in my road map. I think that understanding what I was doing and removing that stumbling block, let me achieve a feeling of peace and calm within myself. That understanding and peace came in incredibly handy as the world was about to become a whirlwind of potential pitfalls.

The Storm of Covid

Covid became and still is a seriously crappy subplot of my story, filled with potential pitfalls. Why do I call it a subplot, because I made a conscious choice not to let it railroad my goal of being healthy? I refuse to see it as the main storyline in my life and give it center stage, even though it has tried to take command during the last year.

Stress and anxiety hit me hard. My bar closed in March 2020, and I was essentially left with nothing to do but twiddle my thumbs at home, and stress over what would happen to my business and my loved ones. I usually have a very slow January and February at the bar. March, specifically St-Patrick's weekend, is where I make my money to break even on the two previous months. I was getting ready for the big parade when the government told all bars to shut their doors. That same day I threw out the fruit and the rest of the garnishes, and everything else stayed as it was with no knowledge as to when I could open up again. I felt overwhelmed. I had this 140-year legacy business that was now in grave peril because I would miss the big March payday. How was I going to ensure its survival and pay my employees? My mind was in overdrive. I thought even if bars do reopen eventually, what if my 92-year old father, who comes to my bar daily, catches Covid there? What if the bar became a super spreader of the disease? Financially I was a mess. My only option was to make some hard decisions. I decided to sell my home and my bar to pay down some of the debt. I had every excuse in the book to play the fool, and allow the subplot to take over and throw my goal to the wayside. Who would blame me for gaining weight or eating poorly? Excuses and emotions abounded at every turn.

This is when my decision not to play the fool paid incredible dividends. Instead of choosing to let go and have my life and diet run amuck, I decided to do a stringent ketogenic diet. I wanted the clarity of having a strict diet. My usual restaurants had closed, and I couldn't afford to take the chance of messing up my food choices by opting for fast food. I also decided to up my walks to two per day and made them longer. Luckily living in the boonies, there were no restrictions on walking outside. This routine minimized my stress because it gave me some control over my life. Control is an incredible feeling, and it surpasses the temporary joy that binge eating used to give me. As the months passed and my house sold, I began to breathe a little easier.

By fall, I decided to stand on a scale and see if my control had created a change in my weight. I looked down at the number and was shocked. I had lost 25 pounds; I weighed in at 190 pounds. That was less than I had weighed in over 45 years. The best feeling was that it didn't feel fleeting, it felt right...

Being fit and healthy has always been touted as important for the longevity of your life. It's not new advice. It's the same advice offered during normal times, with one twist, times are not normal.

Yet, the advice shouldn't change because the times were changing. If anything, during Covid, it has become essential for us all to take care of our health. The CDC published *Coronavirus Disease 2019 Case Surveillance — United States, January 22–May 30, 2020.*

It reported that among COVID-19 cases, the two most common underlying health conditions were cardiovascular disease (32 percent) and diabetes (30 percent). The more I saw how bad metabolic health and Covid interacted, the more it made me wonder that if I hadn't dealt with my diabetes and my obesity. Who knows if I would be around to write this book today?

CONCLUSION

There's an old mantra that goes, "Surround yourself with people who are smarter than you." When I began this quest to fix my health and took up this resolution against sugar, many people thought I couldn't do it. It would lead to nowhere, and I would be fat, sick and on medication for the rest of my life.

One of the best things I did was rely on that old mantra, and tune out all those that didn't believe in me. I surrounded myself with a team of like-minded individuals that were smarter, and had a lot more experience and knowledge. Those like-minded individuals were part of my life through their podcasts, books and articles. They were the team of researchers that I put together; Lustig, Sisson, Attia, Phinney, Volek, Fung and Taubes. I've peppered their names throughout this book, but I can't stress enough how their expertise helped motivate, educate and further my journey along this path.

I binged on their information, using it to harden my resolve. As it got easier, part of me wished I could go back to the fat, unhealthy Rob, and tell him to get started earlier before the need for medication. I know I'm far from alone in the struggle to get a handle on health. It's why I wanted to write this book, to show that it's possible and that it's worth it. I wake up in the morning and I'm happy. As I go outside, walk and take big breaths of air, contentment hits me. Life can be pleasurable and carefree once we remove the shackles that hold us down; the pounds, the cravings, the addictions, and the sugar...

Maybe you're thinking, "Rob, it sounds all too easy, what's the catch?" There is no catch. By taking the first big step, the no added sugar resolution you are one step closer to becoming a metabolic millionaire. Just as the pioneering scientists took the first step in designing the Rosetta Probe, you're designing the new you. This is your mission. Continuing on your journey is priceless!

THE MOST COMMON NAMES FOR SUGAR

1. Dextrose
2. Fructose
3. Galactose
4. Glucose
5. Lactose
6. Maltose
7. Sucrose
8. Beet sugar
9. Brown sugar
10. Cane juice crystals
11. Cane sugar
12. Castor sugar
13. Coconut sugar
14. Confectioner's sugar
15. Corn syrup solids
16. Crystalline fructose
17. Date sugar
18. Demerara sugar

19. Dextrin

20. Diastatic malt

21. Ethyl maltol

22. Florida crystals

23. Golden sugar

24. Glucose syrup solids

25. Grape sugar

26. Icing sugar

27. Maltodextrin

28. Muscovado sugar

29. Panela sugar

30. Raw sugar

31. Sugar (granulated or table)

32. Sucanat

33. Turbinado sugar

34. Yellow sugar

35. Agave Nectar/Syrup

36. Barley malt

37. Blackstrap molasses

38. Brown rice syrup

39. Buttered sugar/buttercream

40. Caramel

41. Carob syrup

42. Corn syrup

43. Evaporated cane juice

44. Fruit juice

45. Fruit juice concentrate

46. Golden syrup

47. High-Fructose Corn Syrup (HFCS)

48. Honey

49. Invert sugar

50. Malt syrup

51. Maple syrup

52. Molasses

53. Rice syrup

54. Refiner's syrup

55. Sorghum syrup

56. Treacle

ACKNOWLEDGEMENTS

I want to thank my friends and family, not so much for their encouragement, but more for their patience in having to listen to me talk about this subject ad nauseam.

I would also like to thank Carolyn Flower and her whole team at Oxygen publishing for making it happen.

BIBLIOGRAPHY

Acton, Rachel, Lana Vanderlee, Erin P. Hobin, David Hammond (2015)

Added sugar in the packaged foods and beverages available at a major Canadian retailer in 2015: a descriptive analysis.

Ahrens, E. H Jr (1992) The Crisis in Clinical Research: Overcoming Institutional Obstacles

Oxford University Press, Oxford.

Ahrens, E.H Jr (1976) The management of hyperlipidemia: whether, rather than how. Ann Intern Med. 85 (1): 87–93

Ahrens, E. H Jr. (1985) The Diet-Heart Question in 1985: Has It Really Been Settled? *Lancet, 1,* 1085–1087, 1085.

Ajala O, English P, Pinkney J (2013) Systematic review and meta-analysis of different dietary approaches to the management of type 2 diabetes. Am J Clin Nutr. 2013;97:505-16.

Andersen CJ , Murphy KE , Fernandez ML (2016) Impact of obesity and metabolic syndrome on immunity. Adv Nutr 2016;7:66–75.

Astrup A, Grunwald G, Melanson E, Saris W, Hill J (2000) The role of low-fat diets in body weight control: a meta-analysis of ad libitum dietary intervention studies. Int J Obes 24(12):1545

Attia Peter (2013) TED: Is the Obesity Crisis Hiding a Bigger Problem? TED.com.

Association of Schools of Public Health (2014) Health Revolutionary: The Life and Work of Ancel Keys. Public Health, Leadership Film.

Avena, Nicole M. Pedro Rada, and Bartley G. Hoebel (2008) Evidence for sugar addiction: Behavioral and neurochemical effects of intermittent, excessive sugar intake. Neurosci Biobehav Rev. 2008; 32(1): 20–39.

Arya, Sumedha (2014) Rethinking Diabetes: An Interview with Dr. Peter Attia. UTMJ, Volume 8 91, Number 1.

Banerjee, Amitav (2018) The Diet-Heart Hypothesis: Changing Perspectives. Miller.

Barnwell, Anna (2018) Secret Sugars: The 56 Different Names for Sugar

Beranty, Richard (2014) The World's Best Fed Army: The K Ration fed millions of American troops and refugees during World War II. WWII History Magazine

Boseley, Sarah (2018) Butter nonsense: the rise of the cholesterol deniers - A group of scientists has been challenging everything we know about cholesterol, saying we should eat fat and stop taking statins. This is not just bad science – it will cost lives, say experts. The Guardian, London, England. p8.

Brouns, F. Overweight and diabetes prevention: is a low-carbohydrate–high-fat diet recommendable? *Eur J Nutr* 57, 1301–1312 (2018). https://doi.org/10.1007/s00394-018-1636-y

Bureau of the Census, *Mortality Statistics 1921. Twenty-Second Annual Report.*

Cai, Jianwen, Boshamer, Cary.C, Stevens, June (2018) Only 12 percent of American adults are metabolically healthy. University of North Carolina, Gillings School of Global Public Health communications.

Canada's obesity rate has doubled since the 1970s. What https://globalnews.ca/news/4456664/obesity-in-canada/

Canada, the Sick - National | Globalnews.ca. https://globalnews.ca/news/4473794/coming-soon-canada-the-sick/

Chen, Y., Wong, S. H. S., Xu, X., Hao, X., Wong, C. K., & Lam, C. W. (2008). Effect of CHO loading patterns on running performance. International Journal of Sports Medicine, 29 (7), 598-606.

Cohen, E et al (2015) Statistical review of US macronutrient consumption data, 1965-2011: Americans have been following dietary guidelines, coincident with the rise in obesity. Nutrition, 31 (5) (2015), pp. 727-732

Cornier, Marc-Andre; Dabelea, Dana ; Hernandez, Teri L.; Lindstrom, Rachel C.; Steig, Amy J.; Stob, Nicole R.; Van Pelt, Rachael E.; Wang, Hong ; Eckel,Robert H. (2008)The Metabolic Syndrome

Cornier MA, Donahoo WT, Pereira R, Gurevich I,
Westergren R, Enerback S, et al.(2005) Insulin sensitivity
determines the effectiveness of dietary macronutrient
composition on weight loss in obese women.
Obes Res. 2005;13(4):703-9.

Cut Down on Saturated Fats (PDF). United States
Department of Health and Human Services.

Davis, Nicola (2017) Is sugar really as addictive as cocaine?
Scientists Row. DC: National Academy.

Demasi M , Lustig R , Malhotra A (2017) The cholesterol and
calorie hypotheses are both dead — it is time to f
ocus on the real culprit: insulin resistance.
Pharmaceutical Journal.

De Walle,Gavin Van, MS, RD (2019)What Are Simple
Sugars? Simple Carbohydrates Explained

Dinicolantonio, James , Wilson, William L. & O'Keefe, James
(2017) Sugar addiction: Is it real? A narrative review.
British Journal of Sports Medicine 52(14)

Doll, Richard & Hill, Austin B (1950) Smoking and
Carcinoma of the Lung; Preliminary Report,"
Br. Med. J., 1950, 2, 739–48.

Dorsey, Patrick. "Mark Sission, 57, shows it's never too
late to get ripped". Retrieved 2018-12-21.

Eating and Activity Guidelines for New Zealand Adults"
(PDF). New Zealand's Ministry of Health.

Ebbeling CB1, Swain JF, Feldman HA, Wong WW, Hachey
DL, Garcia-Lago E, Ludwig DS.JAMA. (2012) Effects

of dietary composition on energy expenditure during weight-loss maintenance. JAMA;307(24):2627-3

Ernst L. Wynder and Evarts A. Graham (1950) Tobacco Smoking as a Possible Etiologic Factor in Bronchogenic Carcinoma; a Study of 684 Proven Cases. *J. Am. Med. Assoc.*, 1950, *143*, 329–36

Evans, Peter (2020) Easy Keto: 70+ Simple and Delicious Ideas. Plum.

Fan Y , Di H , Chen G , et al. (2016) Effects of low carbohydrate diets in individuals with type 2 diabetes: systematic review and meta-analysis. Int. J Clin. Exp. Med 2016;9:11166–74.

Federal Register Proposed Rules - 62 FR 18937 April 17, 1997 - Substances Generally Recognized as Safe".

Finn, Ronald. (1996). Richard MacKarness. British Medical Journal. 312 (7045): 1534.

Forsythe CE , Phinney SD , Fernandez ML , et al. (2008) Comparison of low fat and low carbohydrate diets on circulating fatty acid composition and markers of inflammation. Lipids 2008;43:65–77.doi:10.1007/s11745-007-3132-7

Foster GD , Wyatt HR , Hill JO , et al. (2010) Weight and metabolic outcomes after 2 years on a low-carbohydrate versus low-fat diet: a randomized trial. Ann Intern Med 2010;153:147–57.doi:10.7326/0003-4819-153-3-201008030-00005

Fung, Jason. (2016) The Obesity Code: Unlocking the Secrets of Weight Loss.

Fung, Jason website, the Fasting Method https://thefastingmethod.com/

Little, Jonathan P; Gillen, Jenna B;   Percival, Michael E; Safdar, Adeel;

Tarnopolsky,Mark A; Punthakee, Zubin; Jung, Mary E; Gibala, Martin J (2011)Low-volume high-intensity interval training reduces hyperglycemia and increases muscle mitochondrial capacity in patients with type 2 diabetes DOI: 10.1152/japplphysiol.00921.2011

Lustig, Robert (2013) "Fat Chance: Fructose 2.0", University of California Television, 21 October 2013 (lecture by Lustig updating "Sugar: The Bitter Truth").

Getting the Fats Right! Singapore's Ministry of Health.

Gibney, Elizabeth (2014) Duck-shaped comet could make Rosetta landing more difficult. Nature.

Global Nutrition Policy Review 2016–2017" (2018) World Health Organization. p. 55.

Gower, B & Amy M Goss (2015) A Lower-Carbohydrate, Higher-Fat Diet Reduces Abdominal and Intermuscular Fat and Increases Insulin Sensitivity in Adults at Risk of Type 2 Diabetes. J Nutr. 2015 Jan; 145(1): 177S–183S.

Hales, Graig M., Margaret D. Carroll, Cheryl D. Fryar, and Cynthia L. Ogden (2020) Prevalence of Obesity and Severe Obesity Among Adults: United States, 2017–2018 NCHS Data Brief No. 360, February 2020.

Hall, KD (2017) A review of the carbohydrate-insulin model of obesity. Eur J Clin Nutr (Review). 71 (3): 323–326.

Harcombe, Z, et al. (2015) Evidence from randomised controlled trials did not support the introduction of dietary fat guidelines in 1977 and 1983: a systematic review and meta-analysis.

Harcombe, Z. (2016) Dietary fat guidelines have no evidence base: Where next for public health nutritional advice? Brit. J. of Sports Med. 51.10(2016).

Harcombe, Zoë (2011) Stop Counting Calories & Start Losing Weight. Columbus Publishing.

Harcombe, Zoë (2014) The Harcombe Diet 3-Step Plan. Hodder Paperbacks.

Harland, David M.; Lorenz, Ralph D. (2006). The Current Crop. Space Systems Failures. Springer-Praxis. pp. 149–150.

Haskell, Bob (August 20, 1976). Mad Witch field minus Babbidge, defending champ. [Bangor Daily News.

Hatfield, D. L., Kraemer, W. J., Volek, J. S., Rubin, M. R., Grebien, B., Gómez, A.L., et al. (2006) The effects of carbohydrate loading on repetitive jump squat power performance. Journal of Strength and Conditioning Research, 20 (1), 167-171.

Hawley, J. A., Schabort, E. J., Noakes, T. D., & Dennis, S. C. (1997).Carbohydrate-loading and exercise performance. Sports Medicine, 24 (2), 73-81.

Health Diet. India's Ministry of Health and Family Welfare

Hess, John L. (1978). "Harvard's sugar-pushing nutritionist". *The Saturday Review*. pp. 10–14.

Hyde, Parker N. ; Sapper, Teryn N.; Crabtree, Christopher D.; LaFountain Richard A.; Bowling, Madison L.; Buga, Alex; Fell, Brandon; McSwiney, Fionn T.; Dickerson, Ryan M.; Miller, Vincent J.; Scandling, Debbie; Simonetti, Orlando P.; Phinney, Stephen D.; Kraemer, William J.; King, Sarah A.; Krauss, Ronald M.; Volek, Jeff S.; (2019)Dietary carbohydrate restriction improves metabolic syndrome 1 ,1

Hooper, Lee; Martin, Nicole; Abdelhamid, Asmaa; Davey Smith, George (2015). Reduction in saturated fat intake for cardiovascular disease. Cochrane Database of Systematic Reviews.

Hunt, Caroline Louisa,1917 How to select foods

Hunt,Caroline Louisa, 1916 Food for young children

Insulin Resistance & Prediabetes | NIDDK. https://www.niddk.nih.gov/health-information/diabetes/overview/what-is-diabetes/prediabetes-insulin-resistance

International Sugar Organization website (2020), The Sugar Market

Intermittent Fasting - Your Complete Beginner's Guide. https://www.fitwirr.com/health/tips/intermittent-fasting

Kalm, Leah M.; Semba, Richard D. (2005) They starved so that others be better fed: remembering Ancel Keys and the Minnesota experiment

Kaur J (2014) A comprehensive review on metabolic syndrome. Cardiology Research and Practice. 2014: 1–21

Kearns, Cristin E., Schmidt, Laura A., & Glantz, Stanton A (2016) Sugar Industry and Coronary Heart Disease Research: A Historical Analysis of Internal Industry Documents JAMA Intern Med. 176(11):1680-1685

Keys, A. (1983) From Naples to Seven Countries - A Sentimental Journey. Progress in Biochemical Pharmacology. 19:1–30.

Keys, Ancel, and Joseph T. Anderson. (1954) The Relationship of the Diet to the Development of Atherosclerosis in Man. In a Symposium on Atherosclerosis. Publication 338. Washington,

Keys, Ancel, ed. (1970) Coronary Heart Disease in Seven Countries. Circulation 41 and 42, no. 1 suppl. 1, American Heart Association Monograph No. 29 (April 1970): 1– 211.

Keys, Ancel. (1952) "Human Atherosclerosis and the Diet. Circulation 5, no. 1 (1952): 115– 118.

Keys, Ancel. (1953) Atherosclerosis: A Problem in Newer Public Health. Journal of the Mount Sinai Hospital, New York 20, no. 2 (July– August 1953): 118– 139.

Keys, Ancel. (1956) "The Diet and Development of Coronary Heart Disease." Journal of Chronic Disease 4, 364– 380.

Keys, Ancel. (1980) Seven Countries: A Multivariate Analysis of Death and Coronary Heart Disease. Cambridge, MA: Harvard University Press, 1980.

Keys, Ancel. (1983) "From Naples to Seven Countries—A Sentimental Journey." In Progress in Biochemical Pharmacology 19. Edited by R. J. Hegyeli, 1– 30. Basel, Switzerland: Karger.

Keys, Ancel. (1995) "Mediterranean Diet and Public Health." 173 The Reasons to Embrace the Truth about Fitness American Journal of Clinical Nutrition 61, no. 6 suppl.

Keys, Ancel (1950) The Biology of Human Starvation. Am J Public Health Nations Health. Feb; 41(2): 236–237.

Keys, Ancel (1954) Letters to the Editor. *Lancet, 264,* 37–38.

Keys, Ancel (1956) The Claim of 'Lack of Effect of High Fat Intake on Serum Lipid Levels,'" *Am. J. Clin. Nutr., 4,* 74–76, 75.

Keys, Margaret (1959). Eat Well and Stay Well. Doubleday, New York, New York.

Know More about Fat. Hong Kong's Department of Health.

La Berge Ann F. ; How the Ideology of Low Fat Conquered America (2008) *Journal of the History of Medicine and Allied Sciences*, Volume 63, Issue 2, April 2008, Pages 139–177, doi.org/10.1093/jhmas/jrn001 (2008)

Lee, Sidney, ed. (1897) Rollo, John. Dictionary of National Biography. 49. London: Smith, Elder & Co.

Lunau, Kate (2014) How the sweet killer is fuelling the biggest health crisis of our time. Omni Television.

Lustig, Robert (2014) Sugar is the 'alcohol of the child', yet we let it dominate

Lustig, Robert Website | Promoting global metabolic health .... https://robertlustig.com/

Lustig, Robert (2915) The breakfast table: With kids consuming half their sugar quota first thing, it's no wonder they're getting diabetes and liver disease. We have to fight corporate interests. The Guardian.

Lustig, Robert (2009) Sugar: The Bitter Truth. University of California Television, 26 May uploaded to YouTube 20 July 2009.

Lustig, Robert (2013) Fructose: it's "alcohol without the buzz. Adv Nutr. 4: 226–35.

Lustig, Robert (2014) Fat Chance: The Hidden Truth About Sugar, Obesity and Disease Paperback. Fourth Estate Ltd.

Lynch, Rene (February 28, 2015). Getting primal with Mark Sisson. Los Angeles Times.

Mann, George (1955) Lack of Effect of a High Fat Intake on Serum Lipid Levels. *Am. J. Clin. Nutr.*, *3*, 230–33.

Mann, George V (1993) Coronary Heart Disease: The Dietary Sense and Nonsense. Paul & Co Pub Consortium.

Mann, George V, Shaffer, R.D. & Anderson, R.S. et al (1974) Cardiovascular Disease in the Masai. *J. Atheroscler. Res.*, *4*, 289–312.

Mann, George V, Anne Spoerry, Margarete Gray et al (1972) Atherosclerosis in the Masai," *Am. J. Epidemiol.*, *95*, 26–37.

Mann, George V (1977) Diet-Heart: End of an Era. *N. Engl. J. Med.*, *297*, 644–50.

Mann, George V (1978) Discarding the Diet-Heart Hypothesis. *Nature*, *271*, 500.

Mann G, ed. (1993) Coronary Heart Disease: The Dietary Sense and Nonsense. Janus Publishing Company: London, England.

McDonald, Bruce E.(2004)The Canadian experience: why Canada decided against an upper limit for cholesterol

Meltem Cetin & Selma Sahin (2016) Microparticulate and nanoparticulate drug delivery systems for metformin hydrochloride, Drug Delivery,23:8, 2796-2805, DOI:

Menke, Andy, Sarah Casagrande, Linda Geiss, et al (2015) Prevalence of and Trends in Diabetes Among Adults in the United States, 1988-2012. *AMA*. 2015;314(10):1021-1029. doi:10.1001/jama.2015.10029 https://jamanetwork.com/journals/jama/fullarticle/2434682

Moore, Norman (1900) Willis, Thomas (1621-1675) . In Lee, Sidney (ed.). Dictionary of National Biography. 62. London: Smith, Elder & Co. pp. 25–26.

Mosley, Michael (2013) The Fast Diet: Lose Weight, Stay Healthy, and Live Longer with the Simple Secret of Intermittent Fasting. Atria Books - Simon & Schuster, New York, New York.

Mosley, Michael; Spencer Mimi (2013) The Fast Diet - Revised & Updated: Lose Weight, Stay Healthy, and Live Longer with the Simple Secret of Intermittent Fasting. Atria Books - Simon & Schuster, New York, New York.

Mosley, Michael: Spencer Mimi (2016) The 8-Week Blood Sugar Diet: : How to Beat Diabetes Fast (and Stay Off Medication) Atria Books - Simon & Schuster, New York, New York

Mosley, Michael (2016) *The 8-Week Blood Sugar Diet:* : How to Beat Diabetes Fast (and Stay Off Medication) Atria Books - Simon & Schuster, New York, New York

Muston, Samuel (2013) How many spoonfuls of sugar do you eat without even knowing? The Independent. https://www.independent.co.uk/hei-fi/entertainment/how-many-spoonsful-of-sugar-do-you-eat-without-even-knowing-8438276.htm

Myron, Kevin (2002). Frederick J. Stare, defender of the American diet, died on April 4th, aged 91". *The Economist* (Obituary).

Obesity and overweight - World Health Organization. https://www.who.int/news-room/fact-sheets/detail/obesity-and-overweight

Obesity: 30% of People In the World Are Obese or... https://time.com/4813075/obesity-overweight-weight-loss/

Oddy, Derek J. (2016) The Rise of Obesity in Europe: A Twentieth Century Food History: over effect on body and brain: Heated debate has greeted an article in a medical journal suggesting sugar should be considered an addictive drug, as experts deride the claims as 'absurd'. The Guardian, Society.

O'Connor, Anahad (2016) How the Sugar Industry Shifted Blame to Fat. New York Times, New York, New York.

Olszewski, Todd M.(2015) The Causal Conundrum: The Diet-Heart Debates and the Management of Uncertainty in American Medicine *Journal of the History of Medicine and Allied Sciences*, Volume 70, Issue 2, Pages 218–249

Patterson, Ruth E., et al (2015) Intermittent Fasting and Human Metabolic Health. The Journal of the Academy of Nutrition and Dietetics Volume 115, Issue 8, Pages 1203–1212.

Pedersen, Jan et al. (2012) Response to Ravnskov et al. on saturated fat and CHD", British Journal of Nutrition Perspectives in Medical Research, vol. 6, issue 2.

Peng, Y.D, K Meng, H Q Guan L, Leng R R Zhu B Y Wang et al. (2020) Clinical characteristics and outcomes of 112 cardiovascular disease patients infected by 2019-nCoV DOI: 10.3760/cma.j.cn112148-20200220-00105

Rao, D.P S. Dai, MD, C. Lagacé, D. Krewski (2014) Metabolic syndrome and chronic disease CDIC: Vol 34, No 1, February 2014. https://www.canada.ca/en/public-health/services/reports-publications/health-promotion-chronic-disease-prevention-canada-research-policy-practice/vol-34-no-1-2014/metabolic-syndrome-chronic-disease.html\

Ravnskov, Uffe (2002) A hypothesis out-of-date: The diet–heart idea

Ravnskov, Uffe (2003) The Cholesterol Myths. Gb Pub

Ravnskov, Uffe (2009) Fat and Cholesterol are Good for You. Gb Pub

Richardson S , Hirsch JS , Narasimhan M , et al (2020) Presenting characteristics, comorbidities, and outcomes among 5700 patients hospitalized with COVID-19 in the new York City area. JAMA 2020.

Sackner-Bernstein J , Kanter D , Kaul S (2015) Dietary intervention for overweight and obese adults: comparison of low-carbohydrate and low-fat diets. A Meta-Analysis. PLoS One 2015;10:e0139817.doi:10.1371/journal. pone.0139817

Shai I , Schwarzfuchs D , Henkin Y , et al. (2008) Weight loss with a low-carbohydrate, Mediterranean, or low-fat diet. N Engl J Med 2008;359:229–41.doi:10.1056/ NEJMoa0708681

Sisson, Mark (2009) The Primal Blueprint: Reprogram your genes for effortless weight loss, vibrant health, and boundless energy. Primal Nutrition, Inc.

Sisson, Mark (2019) The Primal BluePrint. Primal Nutrition, Inc. Fourth Edition, New edition.

Sisson, Mark (website) Mark's Daily Apple

Snyder, C. R.; Lopez, Shane J. (2007) Positive Psychology. Sage Publications, Inc.

Statistics Canada (2015) Sugar consumption among Canadians off all ages. Government of Canada, Ottawa, Ontario.

Statistics Canada, 2016 and 2017. Canadian Health Measures Survey. Ottawa.

Statistics Canada, 2007 to 2009. Canadian Health Measures Survey. Ottawa.

Statistics Canada, 2017. Canadian Community Health Survey. Ottawa.

Statistics Canada (2018) Statistics Canada Health Fact Sheet, Ottawa.

Stokes EK , Zambrano LD , Anderson KN , et al. (2020) Coronavirus Disease 2019 Case Surveillance - United States, January 22-May 30, 2020. MMWR Morb Mortal Wkly Rep 2020;69:759–65.

Sumithran, L & Prendergast, E Delbridge, K Purcell, A Shulkes, A Kriketos, J Proietto (2013) Ketosis and Appetite-Mediating Nutrients and Hormones After Weight Loss

Eur J Clin Nutr, 2013 Jul;67(7):759-64.

Taubes G. (2011) The Case Against Sugar, Penguin-Random House, Toronto, Ontario.

Taubes G. (2011) Why we get fat and what to do about it, Random House, Toronto, Ontario.

Taubes, Gary. (2001) "The Soft Science of Dietary Fat." Science. 291, no. 5513 (March 2001): 2536– 2545.

Taubes, Gary. (2002) "What if It's All Been a Big Fat Lie?" New York Times Magazine, July 7, 2002.

Taubes, Gary. (2007) "Do We Really Know What Makes Us Healthy?" New York Times Magazine, September 16, 2007.

Taubes, Gary. (2007) Good Calories, Bad Calories: Fats, Carbs, and the Controversial Science of Diet and Health. New York: Alfred A. Knopf, 2007.

Teicholz, Nina (2016) The Big Fat Surprise: Why Butter, Meat and Cheese Belong in a Healthy Diet, Simon & Schuster.

The Canadian Clinicians for Therapeutic Nutrition website

The Food and Agriculture Organization website, (2021) FAOSTAT data

The Public Health Agency of Canada (2017) Diabetes in Canada. Ottawa,

The Sugar Association website, https://www.sugar.org/sugar/what-is-sugar/

Times Now Digital (2018)Diabetes causes 1 death every 6 seconds: Here's what you can do about this complex disease

Toffler, Alvin (1970) Future Shock. Random House, New York, New York.

Unwin D, Unwin J (2014) Low carbohydrate diet to achieve weight loss and improve HbA1c in type 2 diabetes and pre-diabetes: experience from one general practice. Practical Diabetes 2014;31:76–9.

US Food and Drug Administration. (1993) Everything Added to Food in the United States. Boca Raton, Florida: C.K. Smoley (c/o CRC Press, Inc.).

Vidinsky, Kate (2010) UCSF Lecture on Sugar & Obesity Goes Viral as Experts Confront Health Crisis. University of California, San Francisco, 11 March 2010.

Volek, Jeff S., Matthew Sharman, Ana Gomez, et al. (2004) "Comparison of Energy-Restricted Very Low-Carbohydrate and Low-Fat Diets on Weight Loss and Body Composition in Overweight Men and Women." Nutrition & Metabolism 1, no. 13 (2004): 1– 32.

Volek, Jeff S., Stephen D. Phinney, Cassandra E. Forsythe, et al. (2009) "Carbohydrate Restriction Has a More Favorable Impact on Metabolic Syndrome than a Low Fat Diet." Lipids 44, no. 4 (April 2009): 297– 309.

Volek, S. Jeff (2012) The Art and Science of Low Carbohydrate Performance, Paperback.

Young Lee, Eric D. Berglund, Xinxin Yu, May-Yun Wang, Matthew R. Evans, Philipp E. Scherer, William L. Holland, Maureen J. Charron, Michael G. Roth, and Roger H. Unger (2014) Hyperglycemia in rodent models of type 2 diabetes requires insulin-resistant alpha cells. Proceedings of the National Academy of Sciences, August 2014

Yudkin, J (1957) Diet and Coronary Thrombosis: Hypothesis and Fact. The Lancet, 6987, P155-162.

Yudkin, John (1958) This Slimming Business. London: MacGibbon and Kee

Yudkin, John (1964) The Complete Slimmer. London: MacGibbon and Kee.

Yudkin, John (1972) Pure, White and Deadly: The Problem of Sugar. London: Davis-Poynter.

Waite E (2018) The Struggles of a $40 Million Nutrition Science Crusade. Wired.

Wax, Benjamin; Brown, Stanley P; Webb, Heather E; Kavazis, Andreas N; Kinzey, Steve (2011) Effects of Carbohydrate Supplementation on Force Output and Time to Exhaustion during Static Leg Contractions Superimposed with Electromyostimulation. Journal of Strength and Conditioning Research. 26 (6): 1.

WHO reveals leading causes of death and disability worldwide: 2000-2019 (2020)

Willner, Tamara (2021) Does Saturated Fat Cause Heart Disease?

Wiklund, Olov (2009). Vi talar inte samma språk", Läkartidningen. Retrieved February, 2020.

Wiss, David A.; Avena, Nicole; Rada, Pedro (2018) Sugar Addiction: From Evolution to Revolution, Front Psychiatry. 2018; 9: 545.

Zinn C, Rush A, Johnson R (2018) Assessing the nutrient intake of a low-carbohydrate, high-fat (LCHF) diet: a hypothetical case study design. *BMJ Open* 2018;8:e018846. doi: 10.1136/bmj open-2017-018846.

ABOUT ROBERT ROYCE GALE

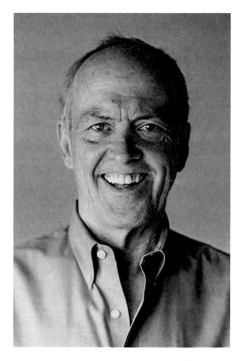

Author Robert Gale lives in picturesque Hudson, Quebec, where he owned and ran the successful historical bar, Chateau du Lac, for 33 years. Recently retired, Robert can now be found working on his popular Facebook page *Sugar Free Resolution*, dedicated to healthy eating and living. He created the blog and this book to share some of the information he learned since he ditched the sugar and reversed his diabetes in 2013.

His weight loss story has been featured in *The Montreal Gazette*, *The Local Journal*, and the online publication, *The Huffington Post*. Robert's hope is to reach as many people as possible to help them lead healthier, happier lives.

Sugar Bitch: How I Ditched the Sugar and Ate my Way Out of Obesity and Type 2 Diabetes is Robert's first book.

For information on Robert and his journey to an optimal life, please visit www.robertroycegale.com